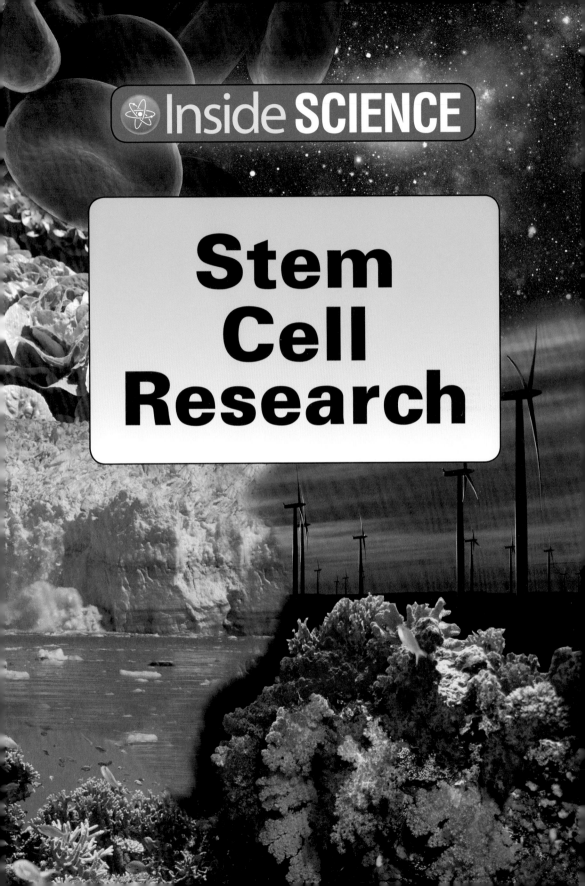

Inside **SCIENCE**

Stem
Cell
Research

Other titles in the *Inside Science* series:

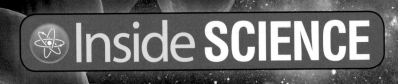

Inside SCIENCE

Stem Cell Research

Hal Marcovitz

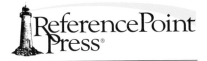

ReferencePoint Press®

San Diego, CA

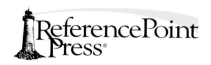

© 2011 ReferencePoint Press, Inc.

For more information, contact:
ReferencePoint Press, Inc.
PO Box 27779
San Diego, CA 92198
www.ReferencePointPress.com

LIBRARY OF CONGRESS CATALOGING-IN-PUBLICATION DATA

Marcovitz, Hal.
  Stem cell research / by Hal Marcovitz.
     p. cm. — (Inside science)
  Includes bibliographical references and index.
  ISBN-13: 978-1-60152-130-9 (hardback)
  ISBN-10: 1-60152-130-8 (hardback)
  1. Stem cells—Research. 2. Embryonic stem cells—Research. I. Title.
  QH588.S83M35 2011
  616'.02774—dc22

                                                                    2010004128

Contents

Foreword

In 2008, when the Yale Project on Climate Change and the George Mason University Center for Climate Change Communication asked Americans, "Do you think that global warming is happening?" 71 percent of those polled—a significant majority—answered "yes." When the poll was repeated in 2010, only 57 percent of respondents said they believed that global warming was happening. Other recent polls have reported a similar shift in public opinion about climate change.

Although respected scientists and scientific organizations worldwide warn that a buildup of greenhouse gases, mainly caused by human activities, is bringing about potentially dangerous and long-term changes in Earth's climate, it appears that doubt is growing among the general public. What happened to bring about this change in attitude over such a short period of time? Climate change skeptics claim that scientists have greatly overstated the degree and the dangers of global warming. Others argue that powerful special interests are minimizing the problem for political gain. Unlike experiments conducted under strictly controlled conditions in a lab or petri dish, scientific theories, facts, and findings on such a critical topic as climate change are often subject to personal, political, and media bias—whether for good or for ill.

At its core, however, scientific research is not about politics or 30-second sound bites. Scientific research is about questions and measurable observations. Science is the process of discovery and the means for developing a better understanding of ourselves and the world around us. Science strives for facts and conclusions unencumbered by bias, distortion, and political sensibilities. Although sometimes the methods and motivations are flawed, science attempts to develop a body of knowledge that can guide decision makers, enhance daily life, and lay a foundation to aid future generations.

The relevance and the implications of scientific research are profound, as members of the National Academy of Sciences point out in the 2009 edition of *On Being a Scientist: A Guide to Responsible Conduct in Research*:

Some scientific results directly affect the health and well-being of individuals, as in the case of clinical trials or toxicological studies. Science also is used by policy makers and voters to make informed decisions on such pressing issues as climate change, stem cell research, and the mitigation of natural hazards. . . . And even when scientific results have no immediate applications—as when research reveals new information about the universe or the fundamental constituents of matter—new knowledge speaks to our sense of wonder and paves the way for future advances.

The *Inside Science* series provides students with a sense of the painstaking work that goes into scientific research—whether its focus is microscopic cells cultured in a lab or planets far beyond the solar system. Each book in the series examines how scientists work and where that work leads them. Sometimes, the results are positive. Such was the case for Edwin McClure, a once-active high school senior diagnosed with multiple sclerosis, a degenerative disease that leads to difficulties with coordination, speech, and mobility. Thanks to stem cell therapy, in 2009 a symptom-free McClure strode across a stage to accept his diploma from Virginia Commonwealth University. In some cases, cutting-edge experimental treatments fail with tragic results. This is what occurred in 1999 when 18-year-old Jesse Gelsinger, born with a rare liver disease, died four days after undergoing a newly developed gene therapy technique. Such failures may temporarily halt research, as happened in the Gelsinger case, to allow for investigation and revision. In this and other instances, however, research resumes, often with renewed determination to find answers and solve problems.

Through clear and vivid narrative, carefully selected anecdotes, and direct quotations each book in the *Inside Science* series reinforces the role of scientific research in advancing knowledge and creating a better world. By developing an understanding of science, the responsibilities of the scientist, and how scientific research affects society, today's students will be better prepared for the critical challenges that await them. As members of the National Academy of Sciences state: "The values on which science is based—including honesty, fairness, collegiality, and openness—serve as guides to action in everyday life as well as in research. These values have helped produce a scientific enterprise of unparalleled usefulness, productivity, and creativity. So long as these values are honored, science—and the society it serves—will prosper."

Important Events in Stem Cell Research

1902
German scientist Hans Spemann conceives of the science of therapeutic cloning but lacks the skills or knowledge of cell structure to perform cloning experiments.

1700s
Rene-Antoine Ferchault de Réaumur, Charles Bonnet, Abraham Trembley, and Lazzaro Spallanzani perform the first experiments examining the regenerative powers of animals.

1895
Valentin Häcker names the cells he finds inside the blastocyst of a crustacean cyclops *stammzelles*, or in English, "stem cells."

1953
Leroy Stevens discovers stem cells in the cancerous tumors in mice; after Stevens transplants the cells into other mice, they, too, develop cancer.

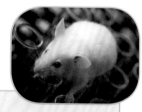

| 1840 | 1880 | 1920 | 1960 |

1859
Charles Darwin publishes *On the Origin of Species*, suggesting that some diseases are inherited from parents.

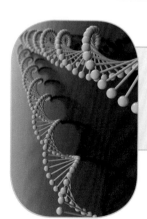

1961
British researcher Francis Crick links DNA to the causes of many diseases when he finds that genetic material provides the instructions for the manufacture of the body's proteins, the chemicals that spark all functions in the body.

1963
Canadian researchers Ernest McCulloch and James Till identify adult stem cells in bone marrow.

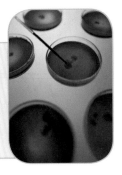

1968
British scientists Robert Evans and Barry Bavister fertilize a human egg through in vitro fertilization; years later, clinics will provide frozen eggs fertilized through the technique to embryonic stem cell researchers.

2002
Scientists at Advanced Cell Technology in Massachusetts employ therapeutic cloning to induce the creation of a blastocyst in a monkey, then harvest stem cells from the embryo.

1998
In separate experiments, James A. Thomson at the University of Wisconsin and John D. Gearhart at Johns Hopkins University create the first human embryonic stem cell lines.

2005
South Korean stem cell researcher Hwang Woo Suk claims to have created active human embryonic stem cell lines through therapeutic cloning; Hwang's work is soon exposed as fraudulent.

1995
At the University of Wisconsin, James A. Thomson creates an embryonic stem cell line with cells he withdrew from blastocysts removed from rhesus monkeys.

1970   **1980**   **1990**   **2000**   **2010**

1981
Biologists at the University of Cambridge in England and the University of California at San Francisco create the first embryonic stem cell lines from cells withdrawn from mice embryos.

2001
Biologists in Haifa, Israel, coax human embryonic stem cells to differentiate into human heart cells.

2009
The U.S. Food and Drug Administration grants permission for the first human trials that involve the transplantation of embryonic stem cells.

2004
Actor Christopher Reeve dies from an infection; paralyzed in a horseback riding accident nine years earlier, Reeve had become an international advocate for the science of stem cell therapy.

2007
Japanese scientist Shinya Yamanaka inserts four genes into ordinary skin cells, turning them into induced pluripotent stem cells.

The Potential of Stem Cell Therapy

Edwin McClure had always been an active and vigorous teenager. He played on his high school football team and had dreams of playing football in college. When he was in high school, though, McClure came down with the symptoms of what he thought was a bad cold or the flu. When the symptoms persisted and affected his eyesight, McClure's mother took him to see an eye doctor. "It was like someone turned down a dimmer switch,"[1] McClure said.

When the physician found nothing wrong with McClure's eyes, he had the teenager undergo a magnetic resonance imaging (MRI) test, which made images of McClure's brain through a process that uses a magnet to energize atoms in human tissue. The MRI test provided McClure with an unfortunate diagnosis: multiple sclerosis (MS).

MS is an autoimmune disease, meaning the disease causes the immune system in the body to attack healthy cells. In the case of MS, the disease targets cells in the brain and spinal cord. Patients who contract MS experience weakness in their muscles and problems with coordination and balance. MS patients often lose their ability to walk; many also lose their vision and feel chronic pain. "I would get fatigued. I couldn't deal with the heat," McClure recalled. "I had really bad balance."[2]

> **autoimmune disease**
>
> A disease in which the body's natural immune system attacks healthy cells; the risk of developing an autoimmune disease is linked to inherited genes, not to exposure to another ill person.

Doctors prescribed drugs to slow McClure's symptoms; the drugs worked at first, but after about two years McClure noticed his eyesight was growing worse. He was suffering from a condition known as optic neuritis, an inflammation of the optic nerve that is common in MS patients. Evidently McClure had built up a resistance to the drugs, meaning they were no longer helping him fight off the symptoms.

Experimental Therapy

As McClure faced the prospect of vision loss as well as the other symptoms of the disease, a doctor suggested an alternative: stem cell therapy. The doctor had learned of a clinical trial at Northwestern University in Chicago, Illinois, that was testing a stem cell–based treatment for MS patients. With nothing to lose, McClure quickly volunteered for the trial.

Red spots surrounded by yellow on the left side of this MRI brain scan mark lesions caused by multiple sclerosis. MS, as the disease is commonly known, affects the brain and spinal cord. Stem cell research offers hope for people with MS.

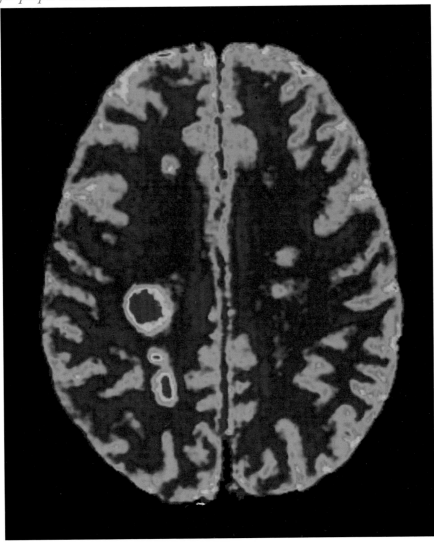

The study of stem cells is more than two centuries old, but only in the past decade or so have researchers made tremendous strides toward curing many horrific diseases and debilitations. Among the diseases that stem cell therapy may help cure are Parkinson's disease, a neurological disorder that manifests itself in slowed and slurred speech, muscle tremors, and rigid muscles, and diabetes, marked by excess sugar in the blood resulting in blurred vision, fatigue, and weight loss and, if left untreated, such complications as seizures, coma, heart disease, and kidney failure. Other conditions that might benefit from stem cell therapy include congestive heart failure, in which the heart grows weak and unable to pump blood to other organs, and Crohn's disease, an inflammation of the intestine that causes pain, vomiting, and weight loss. It is believed that stem cells can also help rebuild damaged tissue, particularly in the spinal cord, helping people whose spines were crushed in accidents walk again.

In simple terms stem cell therapy means using what are known as undifferentiated cells found in the body and growing these into healthy cells, to replace diseased and damaged tissue or make other corrections in a patient's body. Undifferentiated cells have not yet developed into blood cells, bone cells, or cells that make up organs, and therefore they have the ability to grow into virtually any type of cell in the body. At this juncture the research is still highly experimental. According to the National Institutes of Health, an estimated 5 million patients worldwide have received some degree of stem cell therapy. In America no form of stem cell therapy has been approved by the U.S. Food and Drug Administration for the routine treatment of any disease or debilitation.

stem cells

Cells that have not yet grown into specific cells in the body, such as blood cells or skin cells, and are capable of changing into cells that could replace diseased or otherwise damaged cells.

Accepting a Diploma

At the Northwestern University clinical trial, McClure received stem cells drawn from his own bone marrow. Bone marrow is the spongy substance found inside bones where most of the body's blood cells develop. During the trial procedure, doctors withdrew McClure's stem cells and, while they nurtured the cells into duplicating themselves in a lab dish, injected McClure with drugs that destroyed his old immune system. Next they

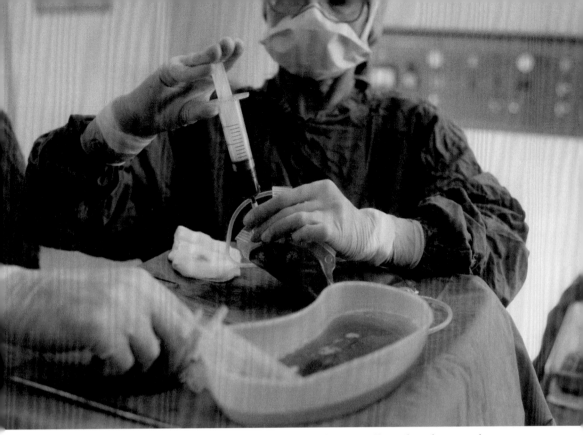

Bone marrow harvested from a patient's pelvis is collected in bags and prepared for transplant surgery. Treatments using stem cells obtained from a patient's own bone marrow are more likely to succeed because there is less risk of rejection.

reinjected McClure with his stem cells, which created a new immune system inside his body. McClure's new immune system was expected to be better able to fight off the MS symptoms. Said Richard Burt, the physician who headed the Northwestern trial, "The concept is that your immune stem cells—your blood stem cells—could be used to regenerate a new immune system in virtually any autoimmune disease."[3]

All indications are that MS is not attacking McClure's nervous system. He said:

> I started to feel improvement while I was in the hospital. I realized that I didn't need my glasses to see. At home my parents noticed that my balance was improving and that I didn't seem as fatigued as before. Honestly, these changes started within the first month after coming home. My life continued to improve. By the third month I was actually going to the YMCA to exercise.[4]

In 2009 McClure received his diploma from Virginia Commonwealth University. He never did get to play on Virginia Commonwealth's football team, but there is no question that the young man who strode onto the stage to accept his diploma was a far healthier person than the teenager who left high school four years earlier—nearly blind, constantly ill, and slowly losing his ability to walk. "I really don't feel like I have multiple sclerosis anymore,"[5] said McClure.

undifferentiated cells

The status of stem cells before they develop into other cells found in the body.

The improvement shown by McClure illustrates the tremendous potential of stem cell therapy. However, other patients have been slower to respond; stem cells have not provided them with the miracle cures that the research has sometimes been said to offer. Their cases help show that despite its promise, stem cell therapy remains a highly experimental process in which doctors are still refining techniques and treatments. Indeed, it is likely to take many more years before doctors fully understand how stem cells work and which diseases they are most likely to cure.

What Are Stem Cells?

The branch of science that holds enormous hope for curing many horrific diseases and debilitations has its roots in some very simple experiments, many conducted more than 200 years ago. That is when scientists first started dissecting tiny animals such as flatworms, roundworms, newts, and zebra fish and finding that these animals possess the ability to regrow parts of their bodies that have been lopped off in the laboratory.

Working in the early years of the eighteenth century, French naturalist Rene-Antoine Ferchault de Réaumur cut off the tip of the claw of a crayfish, then found that it had grown back. A few years later Swiss naturalist Abraham Trembley performed the same experiment on the hydra, which is a tiny aquatic animal about one-half inch (1 cm) in length. No matter where Trembley cut the hydra, it would grow back its missing pieces. Moreover, the pieces that Trembley sliced off the hydra grew their own heads. Another Swiss scientist, Trembley's cousin Charles Bonnet, studied earthworms and drew similar conclusions.

Bonnet shared his work with Italian biologist Lazzaro Spallanzani, who was also studying the regeneration powers of small creatures such as salamanders, snails, slugs, tadpoles, and earthworms. Experimenting on tadpoles, Spallanzani found that if he lopped off the whole tail, the animal would die, but if he sliced off just a small piece, the missing piece would grow back. "If the whole tail, or very near the whole, be cut off, the tadpoles go to the bottom of the water, and there lie down and perish," Spallanzani observed. "But if a lesser part be taken off, not one of them dies, and all without exception recover what they lost."[6]

None of those eighteenth-century scientists understood how body parts could regenerate themselves—all they were able to conclude was that in some animals, lost pieces grow back, whereas in other animals they do not. Nevertheless, de Réaumur, Trembley, Bonnet, and Spallanzani were among the first scientists to witness the power of stem cells.

CHAPTER ONE

Preformation or Epigenesis?

By the nineteenth century the concept of cell differentiation had been accepted by scientists without much agreement on how cells grow into parts of the body. Most theories examined the concepts of preformation and epigenesis. The preformationist view suggests that cell differentiation is decided as the cells are formed. The epigenesist view holds that cells differentiate as the organism forms. The word *epigenesis* has its roots in the Greek words *epi*, which means "upon," and *genesis*, which means "beginning."

A major proponent of the preformationist view was Wilhelm Roux, a German zoologist, who claimed that the fate of cells was determined early in their lives—that only muscle cells could grow into muscle, blood cells into blood, liver cells into livers, eye cells into eyes, and so on. Meanwhile another German biologist, Hans Driesch, argued that cells could grow into any part of the living creature. Driesch had experimented with sea urchins, cutting them apart and then observing how the animals grew back their missing halves. The work of Driesch and other scientists has eventually proved the validity of the epigenesist view.

The Roles of Cells

Cells are regarded as the building blocks of life—every plant and every animal is composed of cells. Humans have trillions. Some living things, such as bacteria and protozoa, are composed of just one cell. Cells are very tiny and can be seen only under the microscope. "The most basic unit of any organism is the cell, the smallest unit of life that can function independently,"[7] says Jay Phelan, a biology professor at the University of California at Los Angeles.

Cells serve two roles: one is structural, the other functional. In their structural role, cells grow into skin, muscles, bones, blood, and the tissue that composes the internal organs, giving these components of the body their physical qualities. In their functional role, cells spark all manner of activities in the body. Cells in the brain, which are known as neurons, create electrical activity that transmits messages to the other parts of the body, instructing the feet to walk, the lungs to draw in air, and the jaw to move during speech. Millions of cells line the retina, which is located in the rear portion of the eye. These are known as rod cells and cone cells, and their jobs are to absorb light that enters the eye and transmit it to the brain, which forms images of what the eye sees. In the abdomen, cells in the pancreas produce insulin, a chemical that helps the body convert sugar into energy.

As these cells form into bone or blood, or as neurons spark electrical activity, they have reached a mature stage of development known as differentiation. Each cell has become specialized, meaning that once it has become a bone cell it cannot change into a blood cell on its own.

Moreover, all cells eventually die. (Anybody who wants to see dead cells need only open the bag of a vacuum cleaner—household dust is composed largely of dead skin cells that have fallen off the body.) However, during their lifetimes cells will duplicate themselves, meaning one blood cell can split into two. Each of those cells will then split, thus maintaining a healthy supply of cells in the body—unless the body is afflicted with a disease or debilitation that prevents the natural act of cell replication. In Parkinson's disease, for example, the symptoms are caused by the death of specific neurons that produce an important chemical known as dopamine, which helps carry the brain's messages from neuron to neuron. In Parkinson's disease patients, these dopamine-producing neurons die much more quickly than the brain can replace them.

Discovery of Stem Cells

Not all cells are differentiated. Some are undifferentiated, meaning they have not yet formed into the cells that compose organ, bone, skin, or strands of hair. These undifferentiated cells are stem cells.

Stem cells received their name in 1895 from German zoologist Valentin Häcker, who found a group of very young cells in the blastocyst of a cyclops, a tiny crustacean similar to a lobster. A blastocyst is an embryo that is no more than a few days old; it consists of just a few hundred cells. Häcker called his discovery *stammzelle*, or in English, "stem cell."

Stem cells can be found in human blastocysts. These stem cells are known as embryonic stem cells. Stem cells can also be found in the bodies of newborns and adults as well. These stem cells are known as adult stem cells and tend to cluster in various places throughout the body. One

blastocyst

A very young embryo, usually just a few days old, that contains no more than 200 or so undifferentiated stem cells.

variety of adult stem cells is found in the blood of the umbilical cord, which is the tube of tissue that feeds nutrients from the mother to a fetus prior to birth. Stem cells found in the umbilical cord are known as cord blood stem cells, and they contain the child's stem cells. Adult stem cells can also be found in fetal tissue that is drawn from aborted fetuses or from fetuses that died through miscarriages.

A colored scanning electron micrograph shows the rod cells (green) and cone cells (blue) of the retina, the thin layer of tissue on the inner eye that makes vision possible. These cells have specific functions: rod cells enable images to be detected and cone cells detect color.

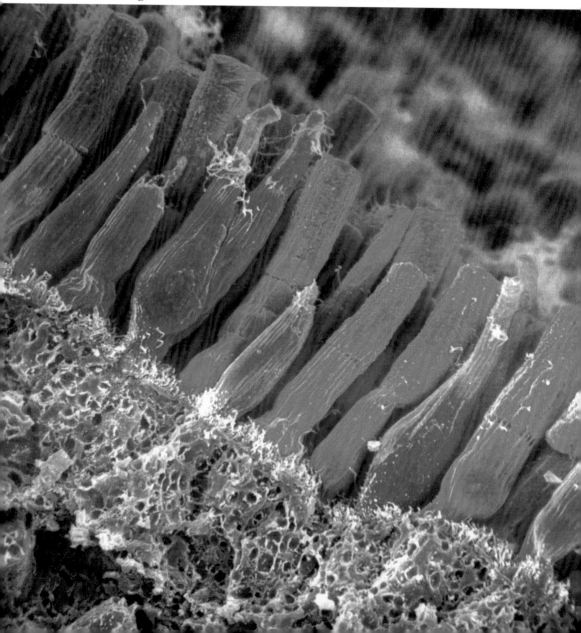

Embryonic stem cells are pluripotent, meaning they are capable of forming into any cell in the body—differentiating into blood cells, bone cells, rod and cone cells, or cells that make up the pancreas or liver. The cells in the blastocyst will develop into all parts of the body, ranging from the hair on a person's head to the toenails on his or her feet.

pluripotent

The ability of stem cells to change into any other cells found in the body.

Most adult stem cells fall short of pluripotency: They are believed to be limited in their ability to change into other cells and are able to grow only into the tissue nearby. In other words, only stem cells that reside in the pancreas can regenerate into new cells in the pancreas. Other adult stem cells, particularly those found in cord blood and certain organs, are considered to be much more capable of changing into other cells. Researchers have found, for example, that adult stem cells drawn out of the liver have been able to replace damaged cells in the kidneys.

When the body is injured, it summons adult stem cells to replace damaged cells, just as the tadpoles summoned stem cells to repair the tips of their tails in Spallanzani's experiments. Says University of Minnesota Medical School stem cell researcher Leo Furcht: "The adult stem cell's ability to regenerate tissue comes from its ability to 'remember' how the tissue was created in the first place. Creating that tissue is the role of the embryonic stem cell, which is found only in embryos."[8]

To differentiate, stem cells receive signals from inside the cell as well as from external influences, all telling them how to change. Each stem cell contains genetic material—deoxyribonucleic acid, or DNA, a molecule that carries the complete blueprint that guides each cell in its role in the development into a living thing. DNA determines the color of a person's hair, whether that person will be thin or

DNA

The molecule deoxyribonucleic acid that contains the code for all the physical components, including diseases, inherited from one's parents.

stout, and, to some degree, the level of the person's intelligence. All of these physical and mental attributes begin at the cell level. Externally stem cells receive signals through chemicals given off by other cells or through physical contact with those cells.

Stem Cell Lines

Stem cells have a remarkable ability to replenish themselves in the body—when they divide, they form new stem cells. They can also keep replenishing themselves in the laboratory. When doctors withdraw stem cells from a blastocyst or from the body of an adult or child, the cells can be cultured in a lab dish to continue dividing and creating millions of new stem cells. These are known as stem cell lines.

Stem cell lines are created by withdrawing the cells from the blastocyst or the body, then inserting them in a dish in a broth known as a culture medium. The culture medium contains various chemical nutrients, similar to the nutrients found in the body, that enhance the growth and division of the cells. Before inserting the cells in the dish, scientists apply biological compounds to the dish surface to provide a sticky surface on which the stem cells adhere; the compounds also help provide the chemical nutrients to the human stem cells. The first stem cell lines were established by coating the dish with a layer of what are known as feeder cells. In most cases these feeder cells were withdrawn from mice. However, mouse feeder cells were eventually discarded because they are believed capable of infecting the stem cells with viruses found in mice. A number of alternatives to using mouse feeder cells have recently been developed: among them are human cells; various proteins, which are chemicals that are generated by human cells; and a compound derived from a small animal in the mollusk family.

As the cells grow and divide, some are removed from the dish and placed in another dish; this is how stem cell lines are maintained. Indeed, just a handful of stem cell lines have produced hundreds of millions of cells and have been sufficient to provide stem cells for hundreds of experiments and trial therapies conducted over a decade or more. The stem cells can be frozen, shipped across the country, and then thawed and employed by scientists working thousands of miles away from the lab where the stem cell line was created.

Getting Stem Cells to Differentiate on Command

Through techniques that have been developed since the 1990s, scientists can induce adult and embryonic stem cells into replacing cells that have died through disease or been damaged through accidents. Getting the cells to differentiate on command is the key. Just injecting them as

Charles Bonnet and Lazzaro Spallanzani

Charles Bonnet and Lazzaro Spallanzani corresponded with each other, sharing their knowledge about regeneration and each adding to the science that would lay the groundwork for stem cell research. Each scientist pursued many other areas of interest, though, adding to other fields of scientific endeavor.

Born in Switzerland in 1720, Bonnet published his findings about the regenerative powers of earthworms at the age of 24. Bonnet's work was cut short by blindness and deafness. Still, he continued to explore science and was eventually drawn into the study of mental health. Bonnet discovered that in some people, hallucinations occur even though the patient may not be mentally ill. This condition is known as Charles Bonnet syndrome. Bonnet died in 1793.

Spallanzani, born in Italy in 1729, also explored fields outside regenerative medicine. He helped disprove the theory of spontaneous generation, which suggests that life can grow from inanimate matter. He was also the first scientist to perform a successful artificial insemination, a process that today is used routinely to breed farm animals and in human reproductive technology. Spallanzani died in 1799.

undifferentiated stem cells into the body can lead to the formation of tumors. This is known as spontaneous differentiation. To carry out so-called directed differentiation, scientists change the environment of the lab dish where the cells are growing. They introduce a broth of proteins and other chemicals, known as growth factors, into the environment of the lab dish to induce the stem cells to grow into specific cells found in the body. These concoctions mimic the conditions under which specific cells are created in the body. The recipe may often include insertion of DNA that promotes cell development, essentially passing on the genetic information from one cell to another. In 2001, for example, the National Institutes of Health reported the success of scientists in repairing the spinal cords of lab rats with embryonic stem cells. The pluripotent stem cells had been subjected to a soup of proteins and chemicals, inducing them to turn into healthy cells in the rats' spinal cords.

Michael Bellomo, an author and executive for a California company that pursues stem cell research, compares the ability of embryonic stem cells to differentiate with the artistic process glassblowers employ to turn shapeless molten glass into vases, bowls, and other finely honed objects. He says:

> The glassblower puffs air into the pipe, creating a bubble, then shapes the [glass] into whatever he or she wants, using everything from wooden paddles with holes to wet paper. Shears can be used to cut the soft glass, or the [glass] can be dipped into molten glass of a contrasting color. This allows the base mass . . . to pick up the properties of the second type of glass.
>
> The parallels to what is being attempted with stem cells are striking. Just as with the molten glass fresh out of the furnace, human embryonic stem cells are pure potential with a minimum of form. Fresh, almost liquid glass can be turned into anything desired. The cells at this state are very similar in that they could potentially, with the right chemical prods, become anything wished for—liver cells, bone cells, any sort of tissue found in the human body.[9]

As differentiation commences, the cells are injected into the body of the patient. Although all stem cell therapies in the United States have been conducted on an experimental basis, many have shown that when stem cells are injected into the body, they replace the cells that have been damaged by disease. Says Furcht, "Creating embryonic-like stem cells and reprogramming adult stem cells to do something other than what they're originally programmed to do makes possible the practice of regenerative medicine—the ability to repair and restore tissues, organs, even limbs damaged by disease or lost to injury."[10]

Dissecting the Swollen Monster

Actually the notion that stem cells can be used to repair damage caused by bad cells and therefore cure disease is relatively new. Although doctors and scientists dating back to Häcker's time suspected that stem cells played a role in regeneration and that this role could probably be put to medical use, it would take decades before scientists realized the full potential of stem cells.

The first important step in determining the importance of stem cells as tools for eradicating disease occurred in 1953 at the Jackson Laboratory in Bar Harbor, Maine, where scientists were at work on a study of cancer under a grant furnished by the tobacco industry—which hoped the lab would produce evidence proving that cigarettes do not cause cancer. Instead, the lab produced a dramatically different finding. Working at the Jackson Laboratory, a young researcher, Leroy Stevens, examined a group of mice that had been exposed to the chemicals found in cigarette tobacco. Stevens soon discovered growths in the testicles of the mice that he suspected were teratomas.

An umbilical cord, still attached to a donated human placenta, is prepared for stem cell harvesting. Stem cells from cord blood can develop into any type of blood cell, a characteristic that makes them desirable for treating numerous illnesses.

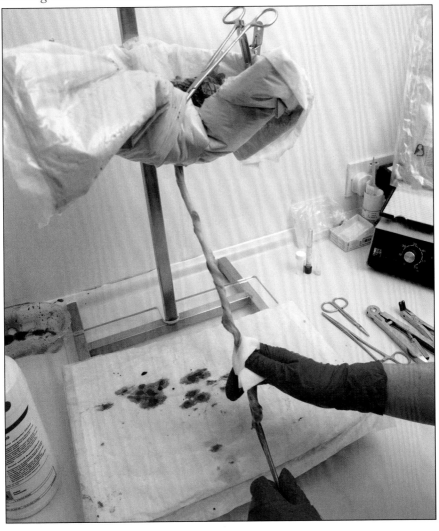

The word *teratoma* is drawn from a Greek word that means "swollen monster." Teratomas have intrigued and puzzled scientists for centuries. Large teratomas surgically removed from humans and animals have included all manner of human tissue and other body parts, including pieces of bone and hair and even human teeth. The rogue cells in teratomas grow on their own, forming parts of the body in places where they should not be forming. Teratomas are, however, more than medical curiosities: They are tumors that are often benign but occasionally cancerous. In cases in which teratomas are discovered in the testicles, as they were in Stevens's lab, the tumors are almost always cancerous.

Stevens dissected one of the mice and examined the cells he found in the teratoma. Some of the cells were twitching and pulsating; Stevens found they resembled the type of cells found in the muscles of the heart. Clearly these cells had differentiated. However Stevens also found other cells that he did not expect to see. These cells seemed to have no function at all; they were simply grouped together, as though they were waiting for instructions. Stevens concluded that these cells were undifferentiated stem cells.

Over the course of several more years, Stevens dissected thousands of mice that had developed teratomas through their exposure to tobacco chemicals and found the same combination of cells in all the specimens. Among the differentiated cells found in the mice were cells that had formed into hair, bone, and blood. Stevens and other Jackson Laboratory scientists withdrew the undifferentiated cells from the teratomas and implanted them into the testicles of

> ### differentiated cells
>
> The status of cells after they have developed into other cells, such as blood cells or brain cells.

healthy mice. Soon these mice developed cancerous teratomas as well—even though they had not been exposed to tobacco-related chemicals. The scientists had used undifferentiated adult stem cells to create a condition in mice that had not existed before.

In this case the Jackson Laboratory scientists had not used stem cells to cure a disease but to create a cancerous condition where the disease had not existed before. Still, Stevens and the other researchers realized the significance of their discovery. By causing cancer to occur in the lab animals, they had witnessed the progression of the disease from its very earliest stages. Essentially they had used stem cells to provide them with vast knowledge of how cancer forms. Said Stevens, "By tracing the testicular teratoma back to its precise origin, we had focused on the very beginning of a cancerous process for the first time in history."[11]

For the next several years, the study of stem cells concentrated on how they developed into cancerous cells, as they had done in the mice in the Jackson Laboratory experiments. Not until the 1990s did scientists realize that stem cells may have other purposes: If stem cells could cause a tumor to form, could they also be used to make a tumor go away?

The Mysteries of Embryonic Stem Cells

F or Kris Gulden life suddenly changed one afternoon in 1996 when, while riding her bicycle, she was struck by a car. Gulden had enjoyed an active life as a police officer in Alexandria, Virginia, but the accident left her paralyzed and confined to a wheelchair with a shattered spinal cord.

Now Gulden teaches high school, and although she says she has a full life, she looks forward to the day when she will walk again. "In my dreams, I still walk. I run, I play basketball and I wear the uniform of the Alexandria Police Department," she says. "When the sun rises each morning, it brings reality with it. I rise to the sight of a wheelchair, yet I rise with the hope that maybe this will be the morning I can move my legs."[12]

The day when Gulden may use her legs again could be more than just a dream. In early 2009 the U.S. Food and Drug Administration (FDA) approved the first clinical trial that employs embryonic stem cells to repair spinal cord injuries. Clinical trials are regarded as the first step toward the widespread use of a therapy to treat an illness or a disability. Trials employ highly experimental techniques and drugs and often must be repeated several times. Indeed, it could take 10 years or more for a drug or similar therapy to move from the clinical trial stage to approval by the FDA for use by the American public.

> **embryonic stem cell**
>
> Stem cell found in the blastocyst; all embryonic stem cells are undifferentiated and pluripotent.

In the years since her accident, Gulden has become an activist for embryonic stem cell therapy and similar experimental procedures. In March 2009, when President Barack Obama signed the executive order authorizing the expenditure of billions of dollars in federal funds to explore embryonic stem cell research, Gulden was invited to the White House to witness the ceremony.

Creating Human Stem Cell Lines

Following the pioneering work by Leroy Stevens and the other Jackson Laboratory scientists in the 1950s, research on stem cells concentrated on mice and other lab animals. A lot of that work focused on identifying and culturing adult stem cells, but in 1981 biologists Martin Evans and Matthew Kaufman at the University of Cambridge in England and Gail R. Martin at the University of California at San Francisco performed independent yet similar experiments on mice. They were able to isolate pluripotent stem cells in blastocysts, withdraw them, and create stem cell lines in laboratory dishes.

During the 1960s and 1970s, a much different type of research was occurring. In 1968 British scientists Robert Evans and Barry Bavister surgically withdrew an unfertilized egg from a woman's body and then, using her husband's sperm, completed the act of fertilization in a lab dish. During the next decade, scientists perfected the procedure and were able to return a fertilized egg to a mother's womb. In 1978 the first baby was born through this process, which is known as in vitro fertilization. (In Latin, *in vitro* means "in the glass.")

Through a microscope a researcher views nerve cells derived from embryonic stem cells. In 2009, the FDA approved the first clinical trial for the use of embryonic stem cells in repairing spinal cord injuries.

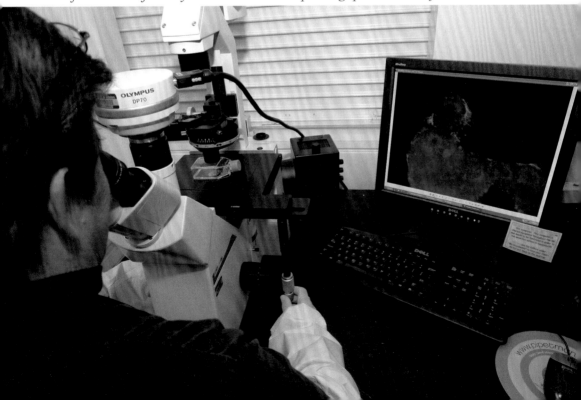

In vitro fertilization has enabled many women who are unable to conceive children naturally to give birth to babies. In America and elsewhere, some 350 in vitro fertilization clinics have been established. Typically a doctor at an in vitro clinic will withdraw several eggs from a patient so that many attempts at fertilization can be made. Successfully fertilized eggs, now in the blastocyst stage, are frozen until they are needed for implanting. After a successful pregnancy, many couples instruct the clinics to discard any remaining embryos.

> **in vitro fertilization**
>
> The medical procedure that enables a doctor to fertilize an egg in a laboratory dish; in Latin, *in vitro* means "in the glass."

Medical Revolution

Following the discoveries by Evans, Kaufman, and Martin, a lot of the cutting-edge work on embryonic stem cell research was performed by biologist James A. Thomson at the University of Wisconsin. In 1995 Thomson created a stem cell line with embryonic stem cells he withdrew from the blastocyst of a rhesus monkey. This was a significant step forward in the research because a rhesus monkey is a primate, and therefore its anatomy is similar to that of other primates, including humans.

Three years later Thomson reported that he created a human embryonic stem cell line by withdrawing stem cells from a blastocyst. The embryos used in Thomson's research were obtained from in vitro fertilization clinics, which, with the permission of the parents, had donated them to the study. Three days after Thomson reported his breakthrough, biologist John D. Gearhart at Johns Hopkins University in Baltimore, Maryland, reported that he also created a human stem cell line. In the Johns Hopkins experiment, the undifferentiated cells were withdrawn from an aborted fetus.

> **gametes**
>
> Also known as germ line cells; cells that will differentiate into cells that compose sperm and eggs only.

The cells employed in Gearhart's experiment are known as germ line cells, or gametes, and would normally go on to differentiate into cells that compose human sperm and eggs. Germ line cells share similar characteristics with embryonic stem cells but while embryonic stem cells are able to grow into lines that include millions of cells, germ cell lines are less able to duplicate, meaning the lines they form are relatively short-lived.

At this time neither Thomson nor Gearhart had developed ways to guide the differentiation of the stem cells they were culturing in their laboratories—they had merely succeeded in making the cells duplicate outside the body. And yet the significance of the discoveries by Gearhart and Thomson was recognized immediately: the technology had potential to help cure many different types of diseases and debilitations. John Fletcher, a bioethicist at the University of Virginia, said embryonic stem cell research would provide hope to people with serious diseases as well as to their family members. "Soon every parent whose child has diabetes or any cell-failure disease is going to be riveted to this research."[13] Added Harold Varmus, former director of the National Institutes of Health (NIH), "This research has the potential to revolutionize the practice of medicine."[14]

Ban on Federal Funding

Others who had been following the research were not as enthusiastic. Conservative Christian religious leaders and others who oppose abortion questioned the ethics and morality of using human embryos as well as cells from aborted fetuses in the research. They argued that even a

 What Is a Blastocyst?

Soon after a human egg is fertilized, it forms a single cell known as a zygote, which then begins to divide. In humans the zygote doubles in size every 12 hours. After about five days, this small mass of cells forms a blastocyst, which is no larger than the period at the end of this sentence. The blastocyst itself is a fluid-filled sphere that will eventually form the placenta, the bag that surrounds the fetus in the mother's womb.

While still in the blastocyst stage, the sphere will grow to include about 100 to 200 undifferentiated cells that cling together. These are embryonic stem cells. At this point in the life of the blastocyst, it includes no features that can be recognized as human; nevertheless, all those stem cells will play a role in the formation of the fetus.

Within a few days the blastocyst will travel down the mother's fallopian tube and implant itself in the uterus. At this stage the blastocyst is known as an embryo. After about eight weeks of development, the embryo is referred to as a fetus.

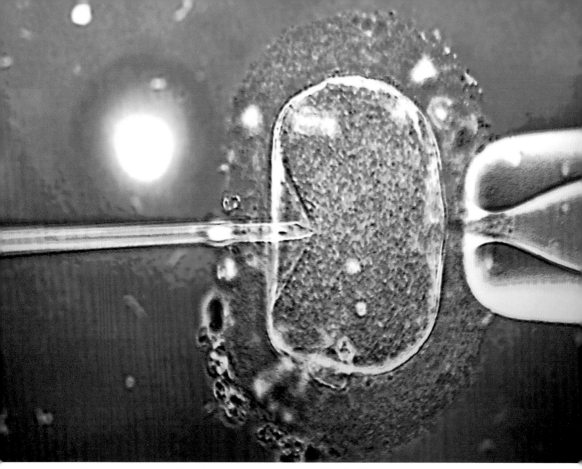

During in vitro fertilization a microneedle (left) injects human sperm into a human egg cell, as seen in this colored scanning electron micrograph. Unused fertilized eggs, or embryos, are a rich source of stem cells.

blastocyst, which is only a few days old and no larger than a tenth of a millimeter, should be viewed as a human life. Removing the cells from the blastocyst would kill the embryo, they argued. "If you view that embryonic fetus as a human being, as we do, then you are using a human being for research,"[15] insisted Edward Furton, director of publications for the National Catholic Bioethicist Center in Boston, Massachusetts.

In America a large proportion of medical research is funded by the federal government, which makes tens of billions of dollars a year available to researchers at university labs as well as labs that have been established by private companies and foundations. Shortly after the 1973 U.S. Supreme Court decision known as *Roe v. Wade* legalized abortion in the United States, Congress passed a law prohibiting federal funding for experiments on fetuses. Lawmakers feared that women would volunteer to have abortions simply to receive payment from laboratories in need of fetal tissue for experimentation. Eventually the U.S. Department of Health and Human Services was given authority to decide whether to fund research on human fetal tissue, but the original ban remained intact through the 1980s and into the 1990s. Indeed, in the labs headed by Gearhart and Thomson, no federal money was used to fund the stem cell research that led to creation of the human embryonic lines.

In the meantime federal rules regarding experimentation on fetal tissue grew even more stringent. In 1995 President Bill Clinton signed a law prohibiting use of federal money for research in which human embryos are destroyed. This law was known as the Dickey-Wicker Amendment because the rules were written by two members of Congress, Jay Dickey of Arkansas and Roger Wicker of Mississippi, both of whom are strongly opposed to abortion.

Three years later though, after Thomson announced his breakthrough using embryos donated by in vitro fertilization clinics, Clinton said he would make federal money available for embryonic stem cell research. Clinton maintained that the Dickey-Wicker Amendment did not apply to the blastocysts that were donated by the in vitro fertilization clinics— the excess embryos were, after all, going to be destroyed anyway. Clinton directed the NIH to begin accepting grant applications.

Ultimately little money would be appropriated. In January 2001 President George W. Bush took office and ordered all consideration by the NIH of stem cell research grant applications frozen until he reassessed the issue. That summer Bush announced that he would permit funding only for projects already underway—by then 64 embryonic stem cell lines had been created at various laboratories. That ban remained in place for the next eight years, cutting off tens of billions of dollars for embryonic stem cell research in America, until the new president took office in 2009 and lifted the ban. Said Obama as he signed the order:

> In recent years, when it comes to stem cell research, rather than furthering discovery, our government has forced what I believe is a false choice between sound science and moral values. In this case, I believe the two are not inconsistent. As a person of faith, I believe we are called to care for each other and work to ease human suffering. I believe we have been given the capacity and will to pursue this research—and the humanity and conscience to do so responsibly.[16]

James A. Thomson

James A. Thomson says he realized the ethical and moral debate his work would stir as his University of Wisconsin laboratory neared completion of its experiment to create the first human embryonic stem cell line. Yet Thomson said he realized that embryonic stem cell research could revolutionize medicine, so he decided to push on with the research. "If human embryonic stem cell research does not make you at least a little bit uncomfortable, you have not thought about it enough," he says. "I thought long and hard about whether I would do it."

Born in 1958 in Oak Park, Illinois, Thomson received undergraduate and graduate degrees from the University of Illinois. Even as a young graduate student, he experimented with stem cells, extracting them from the blastocysts of mice and monkeys. He also received two doctoral degrees from the University of Pennsylvania in veterinary medicine and molecular biology before joining the faculty of the University of Wisconsin.

Before moving on to the study of human embryos, Thomson says he consulted two advisors—law professor Alta Charo and physician Norman Fost. Both urged him to pursue the research. Says Fost, "It is unusual in the history of science for a scientist to really want to think carefully about the ethical implications of his work before he sets out to do it."

Quoted in Gina Kolata, "Man Who Helped Start Stem Cell War May End It," *New York Times*, November 22, 2007, p. 1.

"Biological Pacemakers"

While proponents like Fletcher and Varmus saw tremendous potential in stem cell research to curve such diseases as diabetes, heart failure, and even some cancers by injecting the cells directly into the patients, many researchers took the science in other directions. For example, one area of research that interested many pharmaceutical companies was the use of stem cells to test new drugs.

It often takes years of testing new drugs on humans before the FDA may approve the drugs for widespread distribution to patients. During the early development of new drugs, lab animals are used for testing. It may take several years of successful experimentation on animals before the FDA approves human trials, which may include clinical trials that can last as long as a decade. By using stem cells, though, the drug companies could skip the animal trials and even some of the human trials by testing the drug on cells created specifically to mimic the cells that are affected by the drugs. For example, a drug company developing a medication to treat heart disease could experiment on stem cells that have been differentiated into human heart cells. Therefore the testing could be conducted on human cells without the risk of trying out a new drug on human subjects. Said Thomson, "You could screen 50,000 potential drugs and pick out the three that look most promising."[17]

Embryonic stem cells started showing their capabilities when scientists were able to develop the protein-laden soups that would help them direct differentiation of the cells. One of the first successful differentiation experiments was conducted in 2001 in Haifa, Israel, by researchers at the Technion-Israel Institute of Technology. The researchers were able to differentiate embryonic stem cells into human heart cells. The research held great promise for people suffering from heart disease. In many types of heart disease, the failure of the organ occurs when cells die, which leads to the death of heart tissue. This condition weakens the heart. Therefore, if new cells could be created, diseased tissue could be repaired. Said Lior Gepstein, who headed the study:

> The idea is that if you have a source for heart cells, in the future you can transplant them into a nonfunctioning area [of the heart] and possibly replace the cells. . . . When we have a heart attack, the area of the heart that doesn't receive blood supply actually dies and is replaced by scar tissue.
>
> Because the adult heart doesn't have any regeneration capacity, this area of the heart won't contract any more [to pump blood]. So this can lead to deterioration in heart function and eventually to heart failure.[18]

It did not take long for these experiments to move from the lab dish to trials on animals. In 2004 the Israeli scientists performed a surgical technique on the hearts of 13 live pigs, slowing their heartbeats to mimic heart failure in humans. Next they took human embryonic stem cells that had been differentiated into heart cells and injected them into the hearts of the pigs. The experiment quickly showed results—in 11 of the 13 pigs, the heart rates increased, showing that the stem cells repaired the damage. Essentially the stem cells had acted like pacemakers—the devices implanted in the chests of heart patients that provide mild electrical sparks to keep hearts beating in rhythm. Gepstein cautioned that the experiment had been performed on pigs and was still likely years away from human trials. "It's not like tomorrow people are going to be waiting in line for biological pacemakers, but we are happy to see after a few days a new rhythm arose,"[19] he said.

Repairing Eye Damage

Another study on laboratory animals showed the value of embryonic stem cells in repairing damaged eyes. At Advanced Cell Technology, a private company in Worcester, Massachusetts, researchers were able to differentiate embryonic stem cells into retinal pigment epithelial (RPE) cells. The RPE cells reside in the back of the eye, where they act as housekeepers for the rod and cone cells, clearing those cells of dead tissue and other debris that accumulates in the eye. The loss of RPE cells during middle age is believed to be a major cause of vision loss. Without the cells, the rod and cone cells become clogged with matter that blocks light as it is relayed to the brain. Some 30 million Americans are believed to suffer from this condition.

retinal pigment epithelial cells

Also known as RPE cells, they reside in the back of the eye, where they clear dead cells and other debris that accumulates in the eye; loss of RPE cells during middle age is believed to be a major cause of vision impairment.

For years doctors treated this condition by transplanting mature RPE cells into the eyes of patients, but that type of therapy has often been thwarted by the lack of cells, which are typically withdrawn from eyes donated by people at the time of their deaths. The Advanced Cell Technology experiment showed that if embryonic stem cells could be differentiated into RPE cells, there would be no shortage of cells available for transplant.

Hope for Quadriplegics

One reason the FDA is hesitant to approve embryonic stem cell therapy on humans is the likelihood that the stem cells would turn rogue after implantation, forming cancerous tumors. There were certainly many experiments conducted on animals that showed stem cells could be danger-

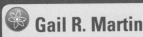 **Gail R. Martin**

When biologist Gail R. Martin developed the process for extracting stem cells from the embryo of a mouse, she did not realize the potential use of her cutting-edge technique. She believed scientists could learn a lot about physical development by studying stem cells, but never envisioned their potential use to cure diseases or repair organs. "Having a big pot of these cells available to produce millions and millions of those little embryolike structures to study, that was clearly a big plus," she says. "But the idea of using them to make new organs really wasn't on the radar screen."

Born in New York City, Martin was working in a lab at the University of California at San Francisco when she first extracted stem cells from a mouse embryo in 1981. In England, biologist Martin Evans performed a similar experiment at about the same time. Using the techniques that Martin and Evans pioneered, University of Wisconsin researcher James Thomson performed the same procedure on a human embryo in 1998, which paved the way for embryonic stem cell research.

Martin, now head of developmental biology at the University of California at San Francisco, says Thomson's work proves how scientists can build on each other's discoveries. "That's something a lot of people don't appreciate—they think, 'Research should be done on my specific disease. But what they don't realize is that cures for those specific diseases may come from basic research for seemingly unrelated areas. What is really going to be important 20 years from now isn't clear."

Quoted in Ulysses Torassa, "Gail Martin: UCSF Scientist Opened Door," *San Francisco Chronicle,* Aug. 10, 2001, p. A-3.

ous. For example, experiments at Indiana University designed to grow new heart cells in mice from human embryonic stem cells indicated that in 3 percent of the cases, the new cells turned cancerous. Also, scientists have raised concerns about the likelihood that the body's immune system would reject the stem cells. Indeed, it is believed that the recipients of embryonic stem cells may have to take antirejection drugs, possibly for the rest of their lives.

Still, many people who suffer from diseases and debilitations seem willing to take the risk. In 1995 American movie star Christopher Reeve, best known for playing Superman, was injured when he fell off a horse.

Reeve's spine was crushed, leaving him a quadriplegic, unable to move his arms and legs. Reeve's plight, and his support for embryonic stem cell research, soon focused attention on the use of stem cells to repair spinal cords.

Early experiments on spinal cords were performed by Gearhart at Johns Hopkins. By 2001 Gearhart had switched his emphasis from germ cells drawn from fetal tissue to working with embryonic stem cells provided by in vitro clinics. Gearhart injected human embryonic stem cells into the spinal cords of lab mice whose spines had been surgically altered to mimic spinal cord injuries. Within a few weeks of the injections, the mice started walking again. "The animals are up and walking," said Gearhart. "It's the first human cells giving rise to repairs in animals."[20] Meanwhile a similar experiment on animals showed how human embryonic stem cells could be differentiated into cells in the pancreases of animals to produce insulin, and another experiment focused on injecting stem cells into the brains of animals to repair brain damage.

Reeve was never able to undergo stem cell treatments. The actor died in 2004 from an infection. Shortly before he died, Reeve told a newspaper interviewer, "If we'd had full government support, full government funding for aggressive research using embryonic stem cells from the moment they were first isolated at the University of Wisconsin in the winter of 1998—I don't think it unreasonable to speculate that we might be in human trials by now."[21]

Five years after Reeve died, the FDA authorized the first human trials employing embryonic stem cells to repair spinal cord injuries. The trial was scheduled to be performed by a private company, Geron Corporation of Menlo Park, California. Participants were expected to receive transplants of embryonic stem cells that had been differentiated into cells that compose the nerves in the spinal cord—the components that send messages to the muscles instructing them to move limbs. Physicians cautioned that the initial dosages would be small and would probably not result in complete recuperation for the paralyzed patients who agreed to the experimental therapy. Nevertheless, University of California at Irvine neuroscientist Hans Keirstead, whose research team developed nerve cells from embryonic stem cells, said, "I would absolutely love to see a quadriplegic regain use of their thumb. That means that person can get out of bed in the morning and operate their own wheelchair. They can type; they can make phone calls."[22]

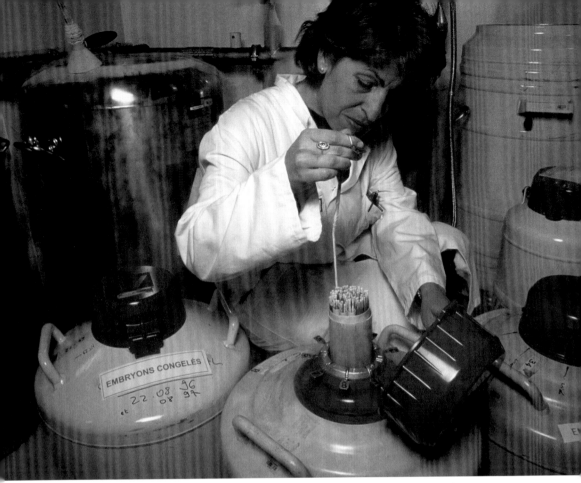

A technician removes frozen embryos from storage in preparation for an in vitro fertilization procedure. After a pregnancy has been successful, many couples instruct in vitro clinics to discard any unused embryos.

Making Human Heart and Eye Cells

In the years since the early achievements in embryonic stem cell research, scientists have pursued a number of procedures that could radically change medicine. In Toronto, Canada, for example, the pioneering work on heart cells conducted at Technion-Israel has been expanded. In 2009 scientists at the McEwen Centre for Regenerative Medicine announced they had grown human heart cells from embryonic stem cells—the researchers actually saw the heart cells pulsating under a microscope. The intention of the Canadian scientists is not to inject the cells directly into a human heart, but to make enough cells to create an actual piece of tissue that would be grafted onto a diseased human heart, repairing the damaged portion of the organ. "It's really reaching out to the cutting edge, to say we can regenerate heart tissue," said Gordon Keller, director of the McEwen Centre. "But given that we can make human heart cells, we have, for the first time, the ability to test this hypothesis."[23]

Meanwhile clinical trials were expected to begin in 2010 assessing the use of embryonic stem cells on patients who suffer from Stargardt's disease, which robs people of much of their eyesight. Stargardt's disease is caused by the deterioration of light-sensitive cells in the back of the eye near the macula, an area of the eye composed of densely packed cone cells. People who suffer from Stargardt's disease have trouble focusing their eyes, meaning they do not clearly see objects straight ahead, such as faces and words printed on a page.

Scientists at Advanced Cell Technology have differentiated embryonic stem cells into cells that are killed by Stargardt's disease. They hope to inject the cells right into the eyes of patients. "It's been over a decade since human embryonic stem cells were first discovered," said Robert Lanza, a researcher for Advanced Cell Technology. "The field desperately needs a big clinical success. After years of research and political debate, we're finally on the verge of showing the potential clinical value of embryonic stem cells."[24]

As human trials commence on embryonic stem cell therapy, public opinion on some of the political issues about the research seems to have shifted. In 2008 a poll conducted by *Time* magazine found that 73 percent of Americans favor embryonic stem cell research and feel the federal government should be supporting the research. Undoubtedly that poll represented the feelings of people who suffer from heart disease, diabetes, spinal cord injuries, Parkinson's disease, and many other illnesses. Indeed, many of them have been waiting a long time for cures that scientists are convinced can be provided through embryonic stem cell therapy.

CHAPTER THREE

Rebuilding Damaged Bodies with Adult Stem Cells

Brent Benson was suffering from congestive heart failure—a condition in which the heart is too weak to pump blood. With little hope for recovery, Benson's doctor told him about a stem cell clinical trial at the University of Utah in Salt Lake City and urged Benson to volunteer. Benson recalls his doctor telling him, "You don't have a thing to lose; you don't have much time left."[25] As a biochemist, the 69-year-old man was well aware of the nature of the trial his doctor had suggested; he was also comfortable with the notion of participating in the experiment. Benson volunteered and was soon accepted into the trial.

Over the course of the next several months, doctors at the University of Utah withdrew stem cells from bone marrow in Benson's body, taking the cells out of a hip bone. Outside his body the cells were differentiated into heart cells, then injected right into his heart. Over the span of several months in 2008 and 2009, Benson received 30 injections of stem cells.

> **bone marrow**
>
> The spongy substance inside bones where most of the cell development of blood occurs.

Since undergoing the therapy Benson has shown vast improvement. The stem cells helped repair the damaged part of his heart: measurements have indicated his heart pumps twice as hard as it did before he received the injections. The most significant evidence of the therapy's success, though, is the simple fact that Benson has already lived much longer than the doctor predicted when he was first advised to seek stem cell therapy. "I've gotten my sense of humor back,"[26] Benson said a year after his treatment.

Benson was not treated with embryonic stem cells but with his own adult stem cells. Adult stem cell therapy has many proponents who believe that therapies similar to the one that extended Benson's life will soon become routine. And unlike embryonic stem cell research, there was never a ban on providing federal money for research projects. The study of adult stem cells has therefore progressed quickly in the past decade, with many therapies moving into the human trial phase. Says James Willerson, president of the Texas Heart Institute, who has pursued similar adult stem cell research, "I believe we will be able to regenerate the whole heart of a human being with stem cells."[27]

> **adult stem cell**
>
> An undifferentiated cell found throughout the body that divides to replace dying cells and repair damaged tissue.

Finding Stem Cells in Bone Marrow

Unlike embryonic stem cells, adult stem cells are not drawn from blastocysts—they are drawn from the patient's own body. This technique avoids the ethical and moral issues involved in extracting stem cells from embryos. In addition, the fact that the donor is usually the patient means that it is unlikely the patient's immune system will react against the cells, rejecting them and making the patient very ill.

As with embryonic stem cells, adult stem cells are undifferentiated. Their primary role is to maintain the health of the body—when skin cells are damaged, for example, undifferentiated stem cells lying dormant nearby go into action, replacing the damaged cells and differentiating into new skin cells.

Adult stem cell research took a great leap forward in 1963 when Canadian scientists Ernest McCulloch and James Till found that bone marrow contains stem cells. McCulloch and Till were not looking for stem cells; rather, they were engaged in research to determine the effects of radiation on living things. This was the era of the Cold War, when the world's superpowers, the United States and former Soviet Union, were amassing huge arsenals of nuclear weapons. At the time, many scientists were exploring what would happen to living things should they be exposed to radiation released during a nuclear attack. The research by McCulloch and Till focused on the effects of radiation on bone marrow, the soft, spongy substance inside bones where most blood cell formation occurs.

While exposing mice to large doses of radiation, McCulloch and Till saw how the toxic effects of radiation destroyed their bone marrow. As part of their experiments, the two Canadians injected healthy bone marrow into the irradiated mice. Later, McCulloch dissected these mice. As Leroy Stevens had seen a few years before, McCulloch saw something under the microscope hc had not expected to see: Clumps of cells had gathered around the spleens of the mice. These were stem cells formerly contained in the bone marrow that had been transplanted into the irradiated mice. Moreover, McCulloch found that some of these cells had already differentiated into blood cells.

The research by McCulloch and Till helped make bone marrow transplants widely available to leukemia patients. Leukemia is a cancer of the blood. In 1956 the first bone marrow transplant was performed on a

🔬 What Are Clinical Trials?

Before a drug or other form of therapy is approved for widespread use in America, it must undergo clinical trials—in other words, volunteers must undergo the therapy under controlled circumstances, monitored closely by physicians. Most clinical trials are sponsored by drug companies, private labs, universities, and foundations that hope to either profit from the therapies or sell the research to others who would make the therapies available to consumers.

Clinical trials require the participation of ill people, but they also need healthy volunteers. According to the National Institutes of Health (NIH), healthy volunteers are recruited for clinical trials because "they provide important medical information to researchers by helping them compare how healthy people differ medically from those who have a specific disease." Volunteers are often compensated for participating, and the NIH requires volunteers to be informed of the risks of undergoing experimental medical therapies.

All clinical trials are monitored by the NIH as well as the U.S. Food and Drug Administration. The NIH maintains a Web site, www.Cinical Trials.gov, that provides the background and status of all current clinical trials, not only in the United States but in other countries as well. In 2010 the NIH reported that more than 83,000 clinical trials were underway in 170 countries. More than 2,800 of those studies focused on adult stem cell therapies.

National Institutes of Health, "Are Clinical Trials for You?" August 27, 2009. www.cc.nih.gov.

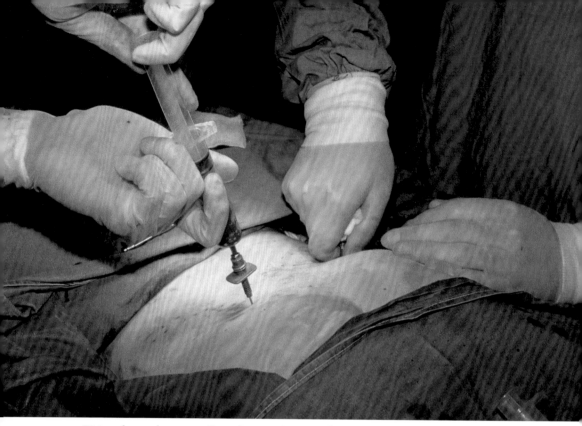

Using large-bore needles, doctors harvest bone marrow from a donor. Following this procedure, the marrow was transplanted into the donor's sister, who had already undergone chemotherapy and other treatments for leukemia.

leukemia patient. The donor was the patient's identical twin. At the time, physicians believed the donor had to be a close genetic match to the patient, due to the fear that the patient's immune system would attack the transplanted bone marrow cells. The experiments by McCulloch and Till helped show that stem cells could be transplanted from one body into another and not be rejected. In 1973 the first bone marrow transplant was performed using a donor who was unrelated to the patient.

Meanwhile, during the 1960s scientists discovered undifferentiated stem cells in the brains of lab rats—an indication that neurons damaged due to diseases or accidents can be repaired by the brain's own stem cells. Over the next several years, scientists made additional discoveries, finding stem cells secreted in other parts of the body. By the 1990s scientists had discovered adult stem cells lying dormant in the human brain, heart, and other organs including skin, blood, bone, teeth, intestines, liver, ovaries, and testicles. Moreover, scientists found that adult stem cells tend to cluster together, in so-called stem cells niches. However, they also discovered that adult stem cells are often few in number and not easy to find—a circumstance that impedes their use in medical procedures.

Stem Cell Soup

Adult stem cells are also believed to be far less capable of changing into other cells than embryonic stem cells. In fact, scientists have designated only a few kinds of adult stem cells as multipotent, meaning they can differentiate into other cells, but to a lesser extent than embryonic stem cells that are pluripotent. Says Leo Furcht:

> All stem cells can renew themselves and develop into specialized cells. For many adult stem cells the potential to regenerate is limited, more or less, to the tissues and organs in which [they reside]. In other words, an adult stem cell from the liver regenerates liver tissue. But some adult stem cells are more versatile; they have more "plasticity" in regenerating body tissue types. Such adult stem cells are multipotent for their potential to regenerate beyond the tissue in which they reside. An adult stem cell from the liver, for example, can be coaxed or reprogrammed to regenerate tissue for the kidney.[28]

Benson's therapy showed that adult stem cells drawn out of his bone marrow could be reprogrammed into heart cells. Additional experiments have shown that adult stem cells found in umbilical cords, bone marrow, and amniotic fluid, which is the fluid surrounding the fetus in the placenta, are multipotent.

The fact that adult stem cells lack the pluripotency of embryonic stem cells does not mean there have not been success stories in adult stem cell therapies. In Japan, for example, scientists have found ways of using adult stem cells to rebuild breast tissue in women who have undergone partial mastectomies.

In breast cancer patients, it often becomes necessary to remove the entire breast—this is known as a radical mastectomy. Some women are

⚛ Adult Stem Cells Versus Embryonic Stem Cells

Conservative Christian leaders and others who oppose embryonic stem cell research argue that since adult stem cell therapy has proved to be so promising, the federal government as well as private donors would do well to focus on adult stem cell therapy. They argue that the same research can be conducted without the moral implications of destroying human embryos. Tony Perkins, president of the Family Research Council, argues:

> Embryonic stem cell research requires dissecting and commoditizing the youngest, most vulnerable humans. . . . Instead of funding more life-destroying experiments, federal funding should go toward life-saving treatments and clinical trials using adult stem cells, which are on the cutting edge of treating patients for diabetes, spinal cord injury, heart disease, multiple sclerosis and other diseases.[*]

Many proponents of embryonic stem cell research counter that there should be room in science for embryonic stem cell research as well as adult stem cell research. They argue that scientists pursuing each type of research should not be regarded as being in competition, nor should either area of research be ranked higher than the other in importance. Says William B. Neaves, president of the Stowers Institute for Medical Research in Kansas City, Missouri: "Those who would pit research with adult stem cells against research with [embryonic] stem cells are trying to mislead laypeople. The overwhelming majority of scientists and physicians in the United States support research with both adult and early stem cells."[†]

[*] Tony Perkins, "Family Research Council President Says NIH Stem Cell Guidelines Ethically Irresponsible," *Medical News*, July 7, 2009. www.news-medical.net.

[†] William B. Neaves, "The Search for Stem Cell Cures," testimony before the Missouri State Senate, Greater Kansas City Chamber of Commerce, January 31, 2005. www.kcchamber.com.

more fortunate: They need not lose their entire breast, but they still have to undergo a partial removal. Nevertheless, a partial mastectomy is still regarded as major surgery and can have a devastating effect on the woman and her body. Using adult stem cells drawn from the patients themselves, University of Tokyo physician Kotaro Yoshimura has augmented the breasts of 39 women who have undergone partial mastectomies.

Yoshimura draws the stem cells out of fat tissue found elsewhere in the woman's body. In fact, the fat is drawn out through the liposuction process, which is a routine procedure performed by cosmetic surgeons to help patients lose weight. The fat is then put into a centrifuge—a machine that spins the fat at a high rate of speed—to separate out a soupy layer of blood that is known to be rich in stem cells.

The cells from this soup are then injected into the women's breasts, along with small doses of fat. After about a month, the breasts of Yoshimura's patients showed growth. This type of research can have a widespread impact on women's health, as an estimated one in eight women in industrialized countries like the United States can be expected to suffer from breast cancer.

Cynthia Fox, a science journalist who has followed Yoshimura's work, says she can see the day when the therapy can be applied to women who have undergone mastectomies. Fox writes:

> If all continues to go well, Yoshimura's stem cell soup, or a version of it, is expected to make a lot of breast cancer patients with partial mastectomies quite happy. And there are few words to describe what such an approach, much more refined, could do for patients who have had full mastectomies. Stem cells may become a cure for one of current cancer therapy's most brutal side effects: disfigurement caused by surgery.[29]

Stem Cell Therapies for Diabetes

Helping breast cancer patients recover from their surgeries is just one of the therapies that has been tried on patients. In Brazil doctors participating in a joint study by the University of São Paulo and Northwestern University have helped diabetics live without daily insulin shots by injecting them with their own stem cells.

Patients who suffer from type 1 diabetes are unable to manufacture insulin on their own. Insulin is an important chemical that helps the body turn sugar into energy. Therefore most type 1 diabetics must receive daily injections of insulin. Diabetes is an autoimmune disease—the body's own immunity attacks the insulin-producing cells in the pancreas.

In the Brazilian trial the stem cells were first harvested from the blood of the patients. The diabetics were then given drugs that killed the white blood cells in their bodies, which in turn destroyed their immune systems. The patients were then injected with their own stem cells, which rebuilt their immunities. In 14 out of the 15 cases, the new immune systems were free of diabetes. "As a research scientist I am always hesitant to speak of a cure, but the initial results have been good and show the importance of conducting more trials,"[30] said Northwestern University physician Richard Burt.

Rebuilding Artery Walls

Another disease in which adult stem cells have been used successfully on human subjects is peripheral artery disease. The condition manifests itself in the clogging and hardening of the arteries. In some patients the condition can lead to heart attacks because blood is shut off from the heart. Other patients experience pain, numbness, and soreness in their fingers and toes because blood is cut off from their extremities. In many cases the disease can lead to amputations. As many as 10 million Americans are believed to suffer from peripheral artery disease.

"Our hypothesis is that people run out of these cells, or they have inadequate supplies, perhaps because of genetic factors," says Keith March, director of vascular biology at Indiana University, which conducted the adult stem cell study on human patients. "As a result, the [cells] can't repair or replace damaged blood vessel cells, and heart disease ensues."[31] In the Indiana University trial, doctors used adult stem cells to rebuild the walls of the damaged blood vessels. During the therapy the stem cells were withdrawn from bone marrow and then injected into the patients' limbs where vessel damage had been detected.

Fifteen patients participated in the trial over the course of 12 months in 2006 and 2007. Most of the participants in the trial were in advanced stages of the disease and facing the prospect of amputation. One of those patients was Ruth Diggs, 78, whose peripheral artery disease was so advanced that she was unable to stand on her own. "I had so much pain," said Diggs. "They were just telling me the only solution for me was to amputate the leg."[32] At the completion of the trial, all of the participants showed improvement—none were required to undergo amputations. "The fact that she has her leg, we are very, very grateful,"[33] said Diggs's daughter, Melvina Jacacki.

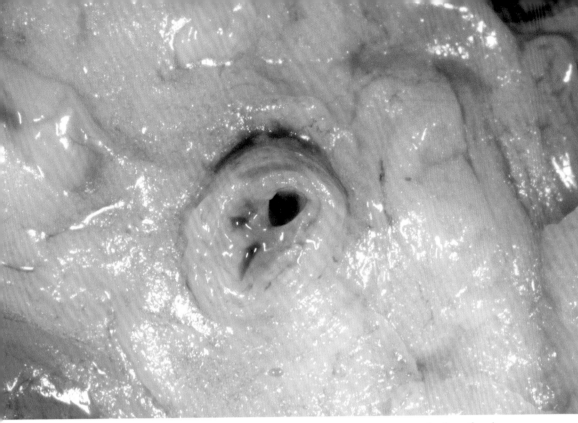

An autopsy reveals a blocked coronary artery, a common and often fatal form of heart disease. Severe blockage prevents oxygenated blood from reaching the heart. Adult stem cells have been used successfully to rebuild the walls of blood vessels damaged by heart disease.

Attacking Congestive Heart Failure

Like Brent Benson, Roger Johnson suffered from congestive heart failure. When the heart fails to pump enough blood, the other organs start to fail. Among the organs most likely to fail are the lungs, which fill with fluid. That was the condition afflicting Johnson, a 57-year-old physician from Manchester, England.

To deal with his heart disease, Johnson underwent triple bypass surgery, a procedure in which doctors graft arteries removed from other parts of his body to bypass three arteries that had become too clogged to function. Also, Johnson had a pacemaker inserted into his chest to help keep his heart beating, and he found himself living on piles of medications. Still, he was growing weaker—doctors estimate that 75 percent of his heart had failed. Johnson could not walk more than half a mile (0.8km) before experiencing exhaustion. He even found himself out of breath as he worked in his garden.

Johnson became a candidate for a heart transplant, but then found himself on a long waiting list for a donor organ. Instead of waiting for the inevitable—complete heart failure—Johnson joined a stem cell trial at London Chest Hospital. He received several treatments of stem cells drawn from his bone marrow and injected into his heart. To reach the heart, doctors threaded a tube, or catheter, into a main artery, entering through his left thigh. After several months of stem cell therapy, Johnson says he feels some improvement and believes his condition has stabilized. "If [stem cell therapy] works, it's probably the only treatment for somebody like myself,"[34] he says.

Johnson was one of 300 patients treated with stem cells in 2006 at London Chest Hospital in what is believed to be one of the largest human stem cell trials to have been undertaken since the therapy moved into the human trial phase. Certainly trials of that size go a long way toward proving the value of adult stem cell research and how it has progressed ahead of embryonic stem cell research. Says David Macauley, chief of the UK Stem Cell Foundation: "We're not sure where the breakthroughs will come. Everybody expects it will come from embryonic stem cells, but the majority of the stuff we are seeing is in the adult stem cell camp."[35]

Building a Better Bioreactor

A lot of the success of adult stem cell therapy is due to the work of biologists who have improved the stem cell lines created with adult stem cells. Embryonic stem cell lines typically last for many years, producing hundreds of millions of cells for research and therapeutic use, but over the years biologists have had a difficult time maintaining the life of adult stem cell lines. In many cases the cells tend to die soon after they are cultured in the laboratory.

Much of the work in improving adult stem cell lines has been accomplished in Canada at the University of Calgary in Alberta, where engineers and biologists worked together to develop better environments in which to grow the cells. For years biologists grew stem cells in what were essentially sealed glass dishes coated with feeder cells, but University of Calgary engineer Leo Behie helped develop a "bioreactor" to grow the stem cells. The bio-

> **bioreactor**
>
> An apparatus in which scientists can enhance the growth of stem cells by adjusting the temperature of the chamber as well as the chemical makeup of the nutrients provided to the cells.

reactor is an enclosed vessel. Biologists can control the environment of the vessel, tweaking the temperature as well as the mixture of oxygen, carbon dioxide, and nitrogen, which are the main ingredients of air. Drug companies have used bioreactors for several years in the development of new pharmaceuticals; Behie headed a project to adapt a bioreactor to culturing stem cells.

By using the bioreactor, biologists have been able to create extensive adult stem cell lines from cells withdrawn from skin, bone marrow, and brain matter and have used the cells in treating Parkinson's disease patients. Said Ivar Mendez, head of neurosurgery at Queen Elizabeth II Health Sciences Centre, "We can send [Behie] a million cells and, four weeks later, we get 300 million back."[36]

Valuable Tools

Adult stem cells may lack the pluripotency of embryonic stem cells, but the efforts by scientists have shown that handicap can be largely overcome, making adult stem cells into valuable tools to combat diseases. Patients like Brent Benson, Ruth Diggs, and Roger Johnson as well as the Brazilian diabetics and the breast cancer patients of Kotaro Yoshimura owe their well-being to the pioneering clinical trials in which they agreed to participate. As for the millions of other people who suffer from heart disease, breast cancer, and peripheral artery disease, they can only stand by and be patient, waiting for the day when adult stem cell therapy will become available to them as well.

Therapeutic Cloning: Altering the DNA of Stem Cells

What would happen if a Parkinson's disease patient received a stem cell transplant in which the cells were genetically altered to treat the disease? In other words, the stem cells injected into the patient would contain a DNA molecule that would correct the conditions causing the Parkinson's symptoms. Theoretically when the genetically altered stem cells enter the body, they will reproduce and eventually replace all the neurons that fail to produce dopamine with healthy, dopamine-producing neurons.

Actually the procedure has already taken place—but not in humans. At Memorial Sloan-Kettering Cancer Center in Los Angeles, California, scientists have cured Parkinson's disease in mice by genetically altering stem cells before they are injected into the brains of the mice.

Moreover, the stem cells used in the study were embryonic but not withdrawn from blastocysts created naturally, such as the type of embryos provided by in vitro fertilization clinics. Instead the blastocysts were created through a process known as somatic cell nuclear transfer (SCNT), or more familiarly, therapeutic cloning. Said Kieran Breen, director of research and development at the Parkinson's Disease Society:

> This is an exciting development, as for the first time, we can see that it may be possible to create a person's own embryonic stem cells to potentially treat their Parkinson's. . . . Stem cell therapy offers great hope for repairing the brain in people with Parkinson's. It may ultimately offer a cure, allowing people to lead a life that is free from the symptoms of Parkinson's.[37]

Bad Proteins

Therapeutic cloning is among the most cutting-edge sectors of stem cell research. It relies on processes and theories that not long ago were mainly fodder for science fiction writers. Today, though, results of SCNT experiments are starting to show that there is real potential for eradicating many diseases by tinkering with the genetic content of stem cells.

The science of therapeutic cloning has its roots in the work of nineteenth-century naturalist Charles Darwin, who wrote that physical characteristics are passed down from generation to generation. Among these characteristics are the color of a person's eyes and hair, whether that person would be tall or short or thin or stout, and, to some degree, a person's level of intelligence. Moreover, Darwin also believed that people inherit diseases such as diabetes, neurological disorders, and cancer from their parents. Darwin was not a physician and therefore did not base his theories on clinical studies; nevertheless over the next several decades many physicians and scientists produced evidence supporting Darwin's assertions that there is an inherited element to many diseases.

Perhaps the most important of these discoveries occurred in 1953 when British scientist Francis Crick and American molecular biologist James Watson unraveled the structure of the DNA molecule, identifying it as a complex and twisted ladder they labeled the double helix. Crick and Watson concluded that DNA carries the genetic code for every characteristic of every plant and animal on earth. In humans DNA is found in virtually every cell of the body.

Moreover, in 1961 Crick established a definite link between DNA and disease when he determined that DNA provides the instructions for the manufacture of proteins, the chemicals that spark all functions of the body. Therefore, if the DNA is faulty, it is likely the proteins produced by the body would be faulty as well, which could cause disease. Given that there are some 100,000

proteins

Chemicals found in the body, numbering about 100,000, that control the functions of all cells.

different proteins manufactured by the human body, it would seem as though there are plenty of opportunities for the body to make bad proteins. In fact, bad proteins have been identified as the cause of diabetes as well as Alzheimer's disease, which creates plaque on people's neurons, robbing them of their memories and other cognitive functions. Another disease attributed to bad proteins is amyotrophic lateral sclerosis, or ALS, which is better known as Lou Gehrig's disease, a progressive, fatal condition that robs people of their cognitive abilities and motor skills.

In many cases the body's immune system attacks the bad proteins and eliminates them before they can do harm, but often the bad proteins overwhelm the body's ability to react to them, resulting in diseases like Alzheimer's and ALS. "Mistakes happen, which is why evolution has endowed cells with sophisticated housekeeping mechanisms to repair or destroy poorly formed proteins before they do harm," write Harvard University professors Peter T. Lansbury and Tom Fagan. "Occasionally, however, a [faulty] protein evades these controls and accumulates in sufficient quantities to clump together and poison or even kill the cell."[38]

Scientists have concluded that there are two ways to treat diseases caused by bad proteins. One way is to treat people with drugs or similar therapies to ease the symptoms caused by the malfunctioning proteins. This method usually does not cure the disease; it simply makes the symptoms more tolerable and prolongs the lives of the patients. The other way is to change the DNA of the cells so they do not make bad proteins. It is believed that this method, which is accomplished through therapeutic cloning, could provide cures.

Cloning Human Cells

In simple terms SCNT involves taking DNA from one cell and inserting it into another cell, where the new DNA will take over and provide new building blocks for that cell. To accomplish this task, scientists employ somatic cells, which make up most tissue in the body. All internal organs, skin, bones, blood, and connective tissue such as muscles are composed of somatic cells, which contain complete copies of the body's DNA. In SCNT the nucleus of a somatic cell is removed and injected into an egg in which the nucleus has been removed. Therefore the DNA from the donor somatic cell has been transferred into an egg.

After receiving the genetic information from the somatic cell, the egg starts to divide, similar to how it would divide after being fertilized by a sperm cell. In this case, though, the new cells have been cloned from the original somatic cell nucleus, rather than created by combining an egg and sperm. Within a few days a blastocyst forms that contains stem cells genetically identical to the original somatic cell.

The first successful attempt to create a human embryo through therapeutic cloning occurred at Advanced Cell Technology in Massachusetts in November 2001. In the experiment 19 donated human eggs, which

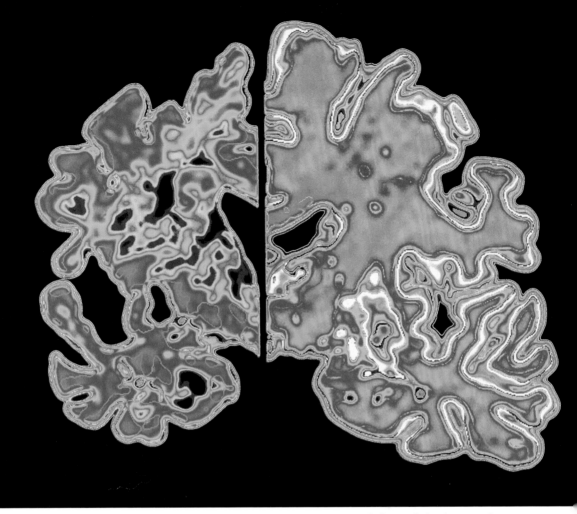

A graphically enhanced image compares a vertical slice of the brain of an Alzheimer's disease patient (left) with a normal brain (right). The diseased portion of the brain (shown in red) is considerably shrunken and the surface is more deeply folded. Efforts to make changes in the genetic content of stem cells may lead to a cure.

had been surgically removed from the female volunteers, were implanted with nuclei from other cells. In 11 of the eggs, the nuclei showed changes, indicating that the new DNA had altered the genetic makeup of the eggs.

Three of the eggs started dividing, creating additional cells. The most successful of those eggs created just six stem cells—not enough to harvest for the creation of stem cell lines. Nevertheless proponents of SCNT saw tremendous potential in what the scientists at Advanced Cell Technology had accomplished—they had induced the creation of embryonic stem cells. "This is the first time cloning technology has been used to grow a tiny ball of cells that can be used as a source of stem cells," said Mary

Can Organs Be Cloned?

Each year, about 5,000 people with failing hearts or other organs die before donor organs become available. The shortage exists because most organs must be harvested from people who have recently died. Living donors can only donate kidneys and portions of their livers.

If stem cells can be cloned through somatic cell nuclear transfer (SCNT) to replace diseased or damaged cells, could they also be developed into complete organs? Scientists at Advanced Cell Technology in Worcester, Massachusetts, have already taken steps toward building entire organs with stem cells. The scientists created cow embryos through SCNT, then implanted the embryos in the mothers' wombs. After a few weeks the researchers surgically removed the kidneys of the fetuses, then nurtured them in the laboratory. A short time later, the kidneys were transplanted into adult cows. After the surgery the cloned kidneys continued to function properly.

This type of experiment is appropriate for animals but would not be permitted in humans. Under law, human fetuses cannot be created for the purpose of providing organs to others. According to Robert Lanza, chief scientific officer for Advanced Cell Technology, the creation of new organs through SCNT would have to occur at a point in which the embryo is still in its blastocyst stage—a scientific accomplishment that is believed to be very far in the future.

Ann Liebert, the publisher of the medical journal *E-Biomed*. "This is an enormous breakthrough that has the potential to be life-saving."[39]

In early 2002 scientists at Advanced Cell Technology announced an even more significant breakthrough: Performing the same SCNT procedure on eggs provided by monkeys, they had induced the eggs to form blastocysts, then produced enough stem cells to create stem cell lines. Moreover, these cells had differentiated into muscle cells, heart cells, fat cells, and dopamine-producing neurons. Some of the cells differentiated in the laboratory, and others were injected into mice, where they further developed. "We let them go wild," said Jose B. Cibelli, vice president for research for Advanced Cell Technology. "They did all these things. We got intestines. We got hair follicles."[40]

And just a short time later, researchers at the Massachusetts Institute of Technology (MIT) announced an important breakthrough of their own. The scientists destroyed the immune system of a mouse, then took a nucleus from a somatic cell found at the tip of the mouse's tail. That nucleus was transferred into an egg, which developed into an embryo and produced stem cells. Those stem cells were then reinjected into the mouse, creating a new immune system for the animal. In other words, the MIT scientists had induced the creation of the mouse's own embryonic stem cells, then used those stem cells to cure a malady in the animal. Said George Q. Daley, the MIT physician who headed the experiment, "This really is a tremendous confluence of very, very challenging technology, wrapping them all together into a model therapy. We are the first to do this all the way."[41]

Research Moves Slowly

Despite the breakthroughs recorded by Advanced Cell Technology and MIT, creating human stem cells through therapeutic cloning techniques has proceeded slowly. Indeed, the science suffered an embarrassing setback in 2005 when a South Korean scientist, Hwang Woo Suk, claimed to have created a robust human embryonic stem cell line using cells produced through the SCNT process. Within a short time Hwang was exposed as a fraud—the doctor claimed he had fabricated the research because he was under intense pressure to produce positive results.

Since Advanced Cell Technology's initial success in creating embryonic stem cells through SCNT, researchers have found that it often takes an enormous number of eggs to perform a successful transfer of a single nucleus. Hwang's fraudulent research paper suggested that he reduced the number of eggs needed to make the transfer from 242 to 17. In some experiments, though, it has taken more than 1,100 donated eggs to make the transfer. Zach Hall, president of the California Institute of Regenerative Medicine, said the scandal may have set the science of SCNT back years. Researchers had hoped to employ Hwang's methods but now have to find other ways to solve the hurdle that requires the use of so many eggs. Hall said, "It's a technological setback and ground we thought we had won must now be re-won."[42]

Hurdles in Therapeutic Cloning

By 2010 researchers were still struggling to create successful human embryonic stem cell lines through therapeutic cloning. Certainly one major handicap to the research is the simple fact that very few laboratories are involved in human SCNT research. Just 10 laboratories in the world are known to be pursuing research into therapeutic cloning. Another handicap faced by scientists exploring SCNT is a lack of government help. Many political leaders are opposed to cloning experiments, fearing that it could lead to reproductive cloning—actually creating life in a lab dish. In reproductive cloning, the blastocyst is not harvested for its stem cells; rather, the embryo is implanted into the womb of a living creature, where it develops as a fetus and eventually is delivered as a baby.

reproductive cloning

Similar to therapeutic cloning, in reproductive cloning the egg created through the transfer is implanted in the womb of a mother, where it grows into a fetus.

Using the techniques of SCNT, scientists have been performing reproductive cloning experiments since the 1950s, starting with frogs and culminating in 1997 with the birth of Dolly, a sheep that was cloned by researchers in Scotland. In the United States many states have passed laws prohibiting the reproductive cloning of humans, but many political leaders insist that the same techniques used to perform therapeutic cloning can be used to accomplish reproductive cloning. Among the abuses that could rise from reproductive cloning of humans is the creation of perfect specimens—exceptional athletes or superintelligent geniuses who owe their talents not to natural evolution, education, and hard work in the classroom or on the athletic field, but to genetic engineering performed in a lab. In 2009 when President Barack Obama lifted the federal government's restrictions on funding embryonic stem cell research, he left in place the restrictions that prevent federal aid to assist therapeutic cloning research.

Getting Results

Despite the many handicaps faced by SCNT researchers, labs have shown results. One issue addressed by the MIT study as well as other experiments was the adaptability of the cloned cell to the recipient's body. When embryonic stem cells are drawn out of blastocysts donated by in vitro fertilization clinics, doctors fear the patient's immune system will attack the stem cells, which is why antirejection drugs are likely to be prescribed to people who undergo embryonic stem cell therapy. In

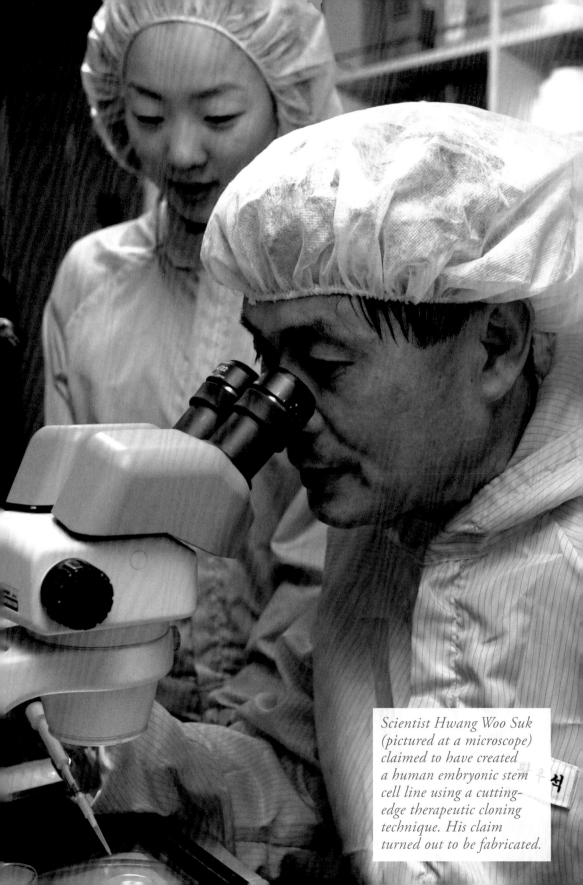

Scientist Hwang Woo Suk (pictured at a microscope) claimed to have created a human embryonic stem cell line using a cutting-edge therapeutic cloning technique. His claim turned out to be fabricated.

The Father of Cloning

The first scientist to propose somatic cell nuclear transfer was German zoologist Hans Spemann. Born in 1869, Spemann was interested in determining the point at which stem cells begin differentiation. He proposed an experiment in which nuclei from progressively changing stem cells are transplanted into female germ line cells, which are cells that eventually form eggs. At some point, he theorized, the stem cell would already be differentiated, and therefore its nucleus would have no effect on the cell to which it was transferred.

He conceived the experiment in 1902, long before scientists possessed the technology to perform a somatic cell nuclear transfer. The first successful cloning experiment would not be accomplished until 1952, when American biologists Robert Briggs and Thomas King performed a somatic cell nuclear transfer on the embryo of a frog, then implanted the embryo into the mother. Later, the mother laid eggs, giving birth to a tadpole created through SCNT.

Spemann is given credit for other important advances in understanding embryos. Spemann tied a hair around the center of a salamander embryo. A short time later two normal salamander embryos were created. This simple experiment disproved the widely held belief that genetic characteristics are lost each time a cell divides. Although the discovery of DNA was still decades in the future, Spemann's experiment showed that each cell in the body contains genetic material.

SCNT, though, it is believed that since the stem cells are genetically linked to the original cell that provided the nucleus for its creation, it is unlikely that the body's immune system would attack these stem cells. Says Leo Furcht: "The SCNT technique produces embryonic cells that are genetically identical to the donor's cells. . . . In therapeutic cloning, stem cells are created through SCNT that can potentially be used to treat the specific illness of the specific patient who donated the DNA."[43]

During the experiment at Memorial Sloan-Kettering, the Parkinson's disease–suffering mice provided the somatic cells that ultimately produced the cloned blastocysts. The stem cells were then harvested and developed in stem cell lines, where they were differentiated into neurons that produced dopamine. The experiment proved the adaptability of the stem cells to the bodies of the recipients—none of the mice rejected its own stem cells. In fact, when the dopamine-producing stem cells were injected into other mice, their immune systems attacked the new cells and killed them. In those mice the Parkinson's symptoms did not improve. "It demonstrated what we suspected all along, that genetically matched tissue works better,"[44] said Viviane Tabar, the lead scientist in the Memorial Sloan-Kettering study.

These results of the Memorial Sloan-Kettering study were followed very closely by advocates for Parkinson's disease sufferers. An estimated 1 million Americans suffer from Parkinson's disease, with 60,000 new cases diagnosed each year. Currently there is no treatment that can slow the progress of the disease, although there are drugs that can help people live with the symptoms.

Among the advocates of using SCNT to cure Parkinson's disease is actor Michael J. Fox, who has been diagnosed with the condition. Fox has established the Michael J. Fox Foundation for Parkinson's Research, contributing more than $4 million to research projects that employ stem cells and therapeutic cloning. "It is the gateway [to a cure]," Fox says of SCNT, "and it's pretty established that it's the gateway to curing and treating a lot of diseases, but especially Parkinson's because it's so specific a problem. If you fix that one thing—if you get the brain to produce dopamine and have the [neurons] accept it in the appropriate measure—you've cured the problem."[45]

Human Trials

Even if stem cells created through therapeutic cloning are not injected into patients, they are still regarded as important tools for doctors that could ultimately provide them with a better understanding of how diseases occur. When a Parkinson's patient provides a somatic cell nucleus to create a stem cell line, the cells in that line contain the genetic information that leads to the disease. Instead of differentiating cells in the line, the researchers can study the disease in its earliest form. Eventually, through a related science known as gene therapy, it is believed that genes that could correct the deficiencies of the patient's DNA can be injected into the patient, thus

genes

Tiny sections of the long chains of DNA in cell nuclei; human DNA has some 23,000 genes, which determine the physical characteristics of each individual.

preventing the Parkinson's symptoms from occurring. Genes are tiny sections of the long chains of DNA in cell nuclei; human DNA has some 23,000 genes. Through gene therapy, defective genes would be replaced by healthy genes, which would then be copied during cell division, eliminating the bad DNA that may have caused disease.

At this point, scientists may be able to cure Parkinson's disease symptoms in mice through SCNT, but humans have yet to undergo therapies that stem from therapeutic cloning. Unlike adult stem cell therapies and embryonic stem cell therapies derived from blastocysts provided by in vitro fertilization clinics, human trials involving SCNT are believed to be several years in the future. One of the reasons human trials are not expected to begin for some time is that the SCNT techniques are so new. Laboratory animals treated with SCNT therapies may not show adverse effects for several years—undoubtedly these animals will be studied closely to see whether adverse effects evolve at some point in the future. For example, in the Memorial Sloan-Kettering Parkinson's study, the researchers announced their findings after gauging the health of the mice for just 11 weeks after they received their stem cell transplants. "They only studied the mice for 11 weeks afterwards, which is not a huge amount of time to see how persistent the results would be,"[46] said Robin Lovell-Badge, a stem cell researcher at the National Institute of Medical Research in Great Britain.

Looking Forward

Still, some SCNT researchers are preparing for the day when the FDA approves their therapies for human trials. In 2009, for example, researchers at the Oregon Health and Science University used the therapeutic cloning process to correct a birth defect in monkeys. The defect is found in a structure of the unfertilized egg known as the mitochondria, which helps provide energy to the egg. If an egg with defective mitochondria is fertilized, the defect can be passed on to offspring who may be born with such diseases as anemia, a blood disorder that saps the strength, as well as many neurological disorders that impede cognitive development.

Using the SCNT process, the Oregon researchers transferred new DNA from eggs afflicted with faulty mitochondria into eggs emptied

> **mitochondria**
>
> Bodies within the cell that provide energy to the cell; defective mitochondria can result in offspring born with anemia and many neurological disorders.

of their DNA but containing healthy mitochondria. After making the transfer, the eggs grew into fetuses. Eventually three healthy baby monkeys were born. Shoukhrat Mitalipov, the lead researcher for the project, predicted that human trials could begin shortly. "Moving to human trials could be very quick, maybe within two or three years," he suggested. "This type of [SCNT] therapy is much closer to clinical application than anything else before."[47]

Despite the slow pace of SCNT research, scientists are convinced the therapy holds great promise for curing Parkinson's disease as well as other afflictions, including diabetes, Alzheimer's disease, and Lou Gehrig's disease. Still, they acknowledge that just a handful of laboratories are pursuing the research while there is no federal aid devoted to the science. They also acknowledge that their research is slowed by the fears expressed by political leaders who believe the therapies could be abused to promote human reproductive cloning. With so many obstacles to overcome, it appears that future breakthroughs in therapeutic cloning may be rare but, certainly, regarded as important breakthroughs nonetheless.

New Advancements, New Challenges

Japanese scientist Shinya Yamanaka found himself conflicted in the stem cell debate. Yamanaka knew the importance of embryonic stem cell research, yet felt haunted by the ethical questions surrounding the destruction of embryos to harvest stem cells. In 1999 Yamanaka, a stem cell researcher at Kyoto University, looked through a microscope at embryos that had been stored at an in vitro fertilization clinic. "When I saw the embryo, I suddenly realized there was such a small difference between it and my daughters. I thought we can't keep destroying embryos in our research. There must be another way."[48]

Instead of withdrawing from stem cell research, Yamanaka dedicated himself to finding a way to make other cells as pluripotent as embryonic stem cells. In 2007 Yamanaka announced his results: By inserting four genes into ordinary human skin cells, he had, in effect, taken them back in time, turning them into pluripotent cells that closely resembled embryonic stem cells.

Yamanaka, as well as scientists at the University of Wisconsin and Harvard University who had been pursuing similar research, labeled these new stem cells induced pluripotent stem cells, or iPS. The breakthrough was welcomed by longtime opponents of embryonic stem cell

induced pluripotent stem cells

Also known as iPS, stem cells created through the process of inserting new genetic material into differentiated cells to turn them into undifferentiated cells.

research, who believed Yamanaka and the others had found a way to uphold the promise of embryonic stem cells without the need to destroy embryos. "Everyone was waiting for this day to come," said Tadeusz Pacholczyk, director of education at the National Catholic Bioethics Center. "You should have a solution here that will address the moral objections that have been percolating for years."[49]

Reprogramming Cells

By making the skin cells pluripotent, Yamanaka and the other scientists had reprogrammed them. This concept is known as transdifferentiation—taking a cell that has already differentiated into one type of cell, then changing its path so that it differentiates into another type of cell. In other words, Yamanaka's research proved cells are like plastic—they can be shaped into other forms.

transdifferentiation

The scientific process of taking a cell that has already differentiated into one type of cell, then changing its path so that it differentiates into another type of cell.

Concerned about using human embryos for the harvesting of stem cells, Japanese scientist Shinya Yamanaka (pictured) searched for a way to make other cells as versatile as embryonic stem cells. His work has led to important breakthroughs in stem cell research.

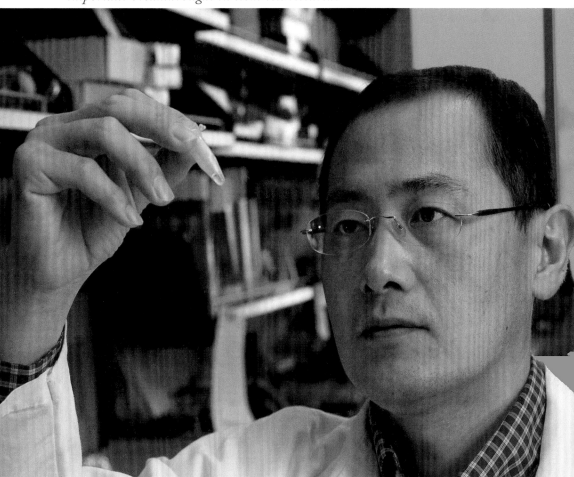

For many years biologists did not think it was possible to change the characteristics of a cell once it had differentiated, but the work by Yamanaka and the others changed their minds. Says Leo Furcht:

> It has been a cardinal rule in developmental biology that tissue-specific . . . cells cannot be reprogrammed. Once a stem cell commits to a specific tissue, it can't go back in time and become a cell that arises from an entirely different [part of the body]. Yet the rapidly growing field of . . . stem cell research is predicated on just that: the "plasticity" of such cells to turn back their biological clocks to when they were stem cells in the embryo.[50]

The key was finding the genes that would instruct the differentiated skin cells to change into undifferentiated stem cells. The human body has 23,000 genes; simply relying on trial and error would have taken years. But Yamanaka had pored through volumes of scientific research on genes and was able to narrow the list to 24 candidates. After experimenting on skin tissue drawn from mice, Yamanaka selected four genes to insert into the human cells. Even so, it took years for Yamanaka as well as the researchers at Harvard and the University of Wisconsin to develop the iPS cells.

Nevertheless, preliminary tests have revealed that the iPS cells and embryonic stem cells harbor similar characteristics. In fact, the researchers have already started growing stem cell lines using the iPS cells. Said James A. Thomson, who headed the iPS research project at the University of Wisconsin, "By any means we test them they are the same as embryonic stem cells."[51]

Concerns About Cancer and Viruses

At this point, though, human trials employing iPS cells are still believed to be years in the future. Indeed, because iPS cells are so new, doctors are leery about injecting them into patients. They want to know if the iPS cells can cause tumors or other harmful effects. One of the genes used in the Kyoto University experiment is known to cause cancer. The fact that the gene was used to reprogram the skin cell does not necessarily mean it will cause cancer in that cell, but at this point doctors do not want to take the chance.

Reprogramming Cells Without Genes

To reprogram differentiated cells to create cells similar to embryonic stem cells, scientists inject them with new genes. The genes then instruct the differentiated cells to revert back to a state before they became mature cells. Scientists at King's College in London, England, and the Universities of Tübingen and Cologne in Germany believe they have found adult cells that can be reprogrammed into embryonic stem cells without the need to inject them with genes.

The source for the adult stem cells are male testicles. Scientists at the three universities found adult stem cells residing among the cells that produce sperm. In a laboratory dish, these cells were then nurtured into taking on the characteristics of embryonic stem cells.

The development could prove to be a dramatic breakthrough. Unlike adult stem cells, the testicular cells can be nurtured into growing into any cell in the body. But if these adult stem cells can be coaxed into acting like embryonic stem cells, it means adult stem cells could be made available to researchers that have otherwise relied on donations of embryos from in vitro fertilization clinics. "The advantage these cells have in comparison to embryonic stem cells is that there is no ethical problem with these cells and that they are natural," said Thomas Skutella, a professor at the Center for Regenerative Biology and Medicine at the University of Tübingen.

Quoted in Seth Borenstein, Associated Press, "Testicular Stem Cells Seem as Versatile as Embryonic Stem Cells," *USA Today*, October 8, 2006. www.usatoday.com.

Another area of concern is the method used to deliver the genes to the skin cells. The gene must be carried into the cell by an organism that can break through the cell wall. To accomplish this task, scientists employ viruses, which are very good at breaking through cell walls. That is how people catch colds and flu—the virus carrying the cold or flu germ attaches itself to the cell, breaks through the cell wall, and deposits its genetic material inside the cell, which in turn causes people to cough, sneeze, feel chills, and run fevers.

To reprogram the cells, Yamanaka and the other iPS researchers employed viruses to carry the genes into the cells. Using viruses as genetic carrier pigeons is a routine method that has been practiced by gene therapy researchers since the 1990s. However, there have been tragic consequences of using viruses to deliver new genes. While most patients receiving gene therapy handle the viruses well, with some not even knowing the viruses have entered their bodies, others have gotten quite sick. In 1999 Jesse Gelsinger, an 18-year-old volunteer in a gene therapy trial, died after his body's immune system was overwhelmed by the virus. Because there are so many unknowns associated with iPS cells, at least for the near future the testing is expected to be confined to laboratory animals.

Still, if iPS cells emerge as a viable therapy, they could provide the type of benefits delivered by both adult and embryonic stem cells with none of the drawbacks of either. Like embryonic stem cells, they would be pluripotent and developed with none of the ethical or moral issues of destroying embryos. And like adult stem cells, they would be drawn from the patient's own body, meaning it is not likely that the cells would be rejected by the immune system. Since they are developed from ordinary skin cells, iPS cells are abundant and easily found, unlike adult stem cells, which are often difficult to locate in the body. "Anyone who is going to suggest that [iPS research] is just a sideshow and that it won't work is wrong,"[52] said Douglas A. Melton, codirector of the Harvard Stem Cell Institute.

Testing Concepts in the Lab

It has not taken long for researchers to start applying the concepts of iPS research to various experimental therapies. At the Whitehead Institute for Biomedical Research in Cambridge, Massachusetts, scientists employed iPS cells to cure sickle-cell anemia in laboratory mice. Sickle-cell anemia is a disease of the blood in which red blood cells form into shapes resembling a sickle, which is an agricultural tool. The sickle-shaped cells are sticky and clump together, cutting off blood flow to organs. In normal blood, red blood cells are shaped like doughnuts and move easily through veins. People who suffer from sickle-cell anemia experience pain, organ damage, and infections because parts of their bodies are starved for blood.

To perform the experiment, the Whitehead Institute scientists extracted skin cells from the mice, in which the sickle cell condition had been artificially induced. Next the mice's skin cells were injected with genes and reprogrammed into stem cells. Those cells were then nurtured into differentiating into cells that produce healthy blood cells free of the disease. Finally those cells were injected into the mice, where they reproduced and soon provided the animals with blood free of sickle-cell anemia.

Meanwhile a joint project by the University of California at Santa Barbara and University College in London, England, reprogrammed skin cells into iPS cells that were differentiated into healthy retinal cells and injected into blind laboratory rats. In the experiment the iPS cells successfully returned vision to the blind animals.

⚛ Mice Born from iPS Cells

Proof that induced pluripotent stem cells, or iPS cells, are truly pluripotent can be found in an experiment performed at three Chinese universities. In 2009 researchers reported that they had cloned mice using iPS cells.

The researchers started out with ordinary mouse skin cells, then injected them with genes to turn them into embryonic stem cells. The nuclei from those cells were then transferred into mouse eggs through the somatic cell nuclear transfer procedure. Finally the eggs were implanted in female mice.

The three universities reported 27 live births. Some of the mouse pups died after two days, and some displayed physical handicaps. Nevertheless, 12 of the mice were deemed to be completely healthy. Those mice were eventually mated with other mice and produced offspring. According to the researchers, there are now hundreds of second- and third-generation mice born from the original 12 that were cloned from iPS cells.

Time magazine placed the Chinese experiment on its list of the top 10 medical breakthroughs for 2009. Said the magazine, "Breeding an entire mouse that is itself capable of reproducing—as the mice did in . . . the Chinese labs—is a strong sign that iPS cells may be as useful as embryonic stem cells for a potential source of treatments for disease."

Alice Park, "Stem-Cell-Created Mice," *Time*, December 8, 2009. www.time.com/time.

Experiments Show Promise

All of these experiments are, of course, still in trial phases involving laboratory animals, but reprogrammed iPS cells may even start showing benefits before they are deemed safe to inject into human patients. As with cells created through SCNT, scientists believe iPS cells can provide keys to the formation of certain diseases. At Harvard, scientists have created iPS cell lines from skin drawn from patients who suffer from diabetes, Lou Gehrig's disease, Parkinson's disease, and other ailments. These skin cells have been reprogrammed into stem cells but still possess the DNA of the donors. Now scientists hope to watch how the cells differentiate and grow, giving them the opportunity to study their genetic makeup to see how the diseases that afflict the donors develop from their earliest stages. Therefore iPS cell lines can enable doctors to watch how diseases may affect cellular development years before the symptoms manifest themselves in patients. Says Melton: "There is a good reason we don't have treatments for diseases like Parkinson's. That's because the only way science can study them is to wait until a patient appears in the office with symptoms. The cause could be long gone by then, and you're just seeing the end stages."[53]

At Harvard, Melton is also exploring further development of iPS cells that would require them to be only partially reprogrammed. This area of research could help provide relief for diabetics. The disease is caused when cells in the pancreas fail to produce insulin. Certainly many research projects are pursuing diabetes cures by employing stem cells that would be coaxed into becoming healthy, insulin-producing cells in the pancreas. On the other hand, Melton suggests, why not take cells that are already in the pancreas and simply reprogram them to start producing insulin? At the Harvard Stem Cell Institute, Melton and his colleagues have already reprogrammed cells drawn from the pancreases of diabetic mice, enabling the cells to produce insulin. "The idea is that you can view all cells, not just stem cells, as a potential therapeutic opportunity," says David Scadden, codirector of the Harvard Stem Cell Institute. "Every cell can be your source."[54]

Some of those cells can be found in human fat. Early experiments have found that fat cells can be converted into iPS cells much more quickly than ordinary skin cells and that they grow in more abundance than stem cells created from skin cells, giving doctors more cells with which to work. "We can get iPS colonies, basically, in about 16 days, compared to 28 days to 32 days using [skin]," said Joseph Wu, a stem cell researcher at Stanford University in California, where the experiments on fat cells were conducted. "And if you count the number of colonies in [skin] versus fat, we get about 20 times more the number of iPS colonies [in fat]."[55]

As with iPS cells reprogrammed from skin cells, these cells would be provided by the patients themselves, and therefore there is little chance that the cells would be rejected by the patients' immune systems. "Even if you're in great shape, there is still enough fat to be harvested from the vast majority of patients,"[56] said Michael Longaker, who headed the study at Stanford. Similar to the breast augmentation therapies performed by Yoshimura at the University of Tokyo, the Stanford study employed human fat drawn out of the bodies of people who had undergone liposuction.

Drawing Cells from Fetal Tissue

As the possibilities of iPS cells are explored, stem cell researchers are refining other cutting-edge techniques they hope will provide cures for diseases. One highly controversial form of research involves the use of fetal tissue to provide adult stem cells. Fetal tissue is drawn from aborted fetuses or through miscarriages of fetuses that are no more than 15 weeks old. The research is opposed by anti-abortion groups. Nevertheless, biologists have found evidence that fetal tissue is rich in adult stem cells that have proved to be much more capable of changing into other cells than adult stem cells available from other sources. Fetal cells are considered valuable for stem cell research because of their capacity to rapidly divide, grow, and adapt to new environments. Moreover, fetal cells are less likely to be rejected by the immune systems of the patients.

> **fetal tissue**
>
> Tissue obtained from aborted fetuses or miscarriages; fetal tissue is usually rich in adult stem cells that can differentiate into many other types of cells.

A recent study by the University of Wisconsin employed stem cells drawn from fetal tissue to reverse the symptoms of Lou Gehrig's disease in laboratory rats. Lou Gehrig's disease is so-named because it afflicted one of the greatest baseball players of the twentieth century, Lou Gehrig

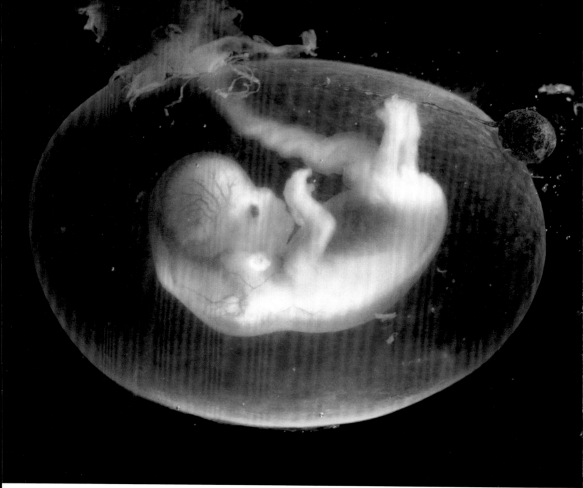

As the human embryo becomes a fetus, around week eight, the eye and limbs are visible and the kidneys, liver, brain, and lungs are beginning to function. The discovery that fetal tissue is rich with adult stem cells has led to controversial research using tissue from aborted fetuses.

of the New York Yankees. The disease, formally known as amyotrophic lateral sclerosis, or ALS, kills nerve cells in the brain and spinal cord, leading to a loss of cognitive abilities and the ability to walk and perform other tasks. In most cases the disease is fatal.

During the University of Wisconsin study, scientists inserted genes into fetal tissue stem cells to produce a protein known to protect brain cells and enhance their development. It is believed ALS patients lack this protein. These genetically altered stem cells were then injected into the spinal cords of rats with ALS. Once in the rats' bodies, the cells attached themselves to nerve cells and started pumping out the protein. In the University of Wisconsin experiment, about 30 percent of the nerve cells that received the protein survived, indicating that the therapy holds great promise for at least slowing the progression of ALS.

Searching for a Cure in China

As with many forms of experimental stem cell therapy, human trials in the United States are believed to be years away. However, some ALS sufferers feel they cannot wait that long and have sought similar treatments outside of the country, where government controls over medicine are less stringent. Kim Allen, a 49-year-old ALS patient from Sioux City, Iowa, felt she had no other choice. Her symptoms had been growing progressively worse—she had been losing her ability to move her hands and feet and communicate with others. In 2005 doctors told her she had no more than 18 months to live. When Allen heard that physicians in China were treating ALS patients with stem cells drawn from fetal tissue, Allen made the decision to undergo the therapy. "This was the only choice I had," says Allen. "I was determined to come here to see if it would help me."[57]

At the Chinese clinic, doctors drilled two tiny holes in her skull, then injected her brain with 2 million cells cultured from fetal tissue. Days after undergoing the therapy, Allen says she noticed improvement. "I can smack my lips for the first time in eight months. It sounds like a simple thing, but when it's something you can't do. . . ."[58]

Back in the United States, physicians are wary of the Chinese ALS treatments, arguing that they are conducted without first undergoing clinical trials that would show possible adverse effects. Still, since many ALS patients regard the disease as a death sentence, they feel they have little to lose by undergoing the treatments. "I wanted to be able to talk better and walk better and get my strength back," Allen says. "I lost a brother to ALS 15 years ago, and at that time they didn't have anything like this."[59]

Stem Cells from Umbilical Cord Blood

In addition to fetal tissue, another rich source of adult stem cells is blood drawn from umbilical cords. At the University of Minnesota, doctors used stem cells found in cord blood to reverse the effects of stroke in lab rats. A stroke occurs when the blood supply to the brain is interrupted, killing neurons. Strokes can cause severe neurological damage; patients can lose their ability to speak and use their arms and legs. Strokes can also be fatal. In the University of Minnesota experiment, strokes were induced in the rats, which then received injections of human stem cells drawn from cord blood.

Meanwhile other cord blood therapies have moved into the human trial phase. Some 70 diseases, mostly anemia and cancers of the blood, have been treated on an experimental basis with stem cells drawn from cord blood. "[Cord blood stem cells] can be used to replace failed blood cells,"[60] says Kristine Gebbie, a professor of nursing at Columbia University in New York City.

cord blood stem cells

Stem cells obtained from the blood found in the umbilical cord, which provides the fetus with nutrients from the mother; cord blood stem cells have the ability to differentiate into many different types of cells.

Dramatic Leaps

More than 250 years ago, Abraham Trembley, Charles Bonnet, Lazzaro Spallanzani, and other pioneers watched as tiny animals lost parts of their bodies but miraculously grew them back. Those eighteenth-century scientists did not understand that they were watching stem cells at work. In the years since those pioneers conducted their studies, particularly in the past two decades, scientists have realized the full potential of stem cells—that they can be employed to combat diseases and disabilities.

In recent years stem cell research has made many dramatic leaps. New information has emerged about adult stem cells, making them more useful than originally believed. Despite the ethical issues surrounding embryonic stem cells, most scientists are in agreement that they hold tremendous potential for revolutionizing medicine. And the recent developments involving somatic cell nuclear transfer as well as induced pluripotent stem cells illustrates how new avenues are constantly being opened in stem cell research. Indeed, the fact that iPS cells can be reprogrammed into pluripotent cells with cells that have already differentiated has shocked many scientists. Faced with this new evidence, they have dismissed their long-held beliefs that once a cell becomes a skin cell it stays a skin cell for the rest of its life.

These types of revelations arc not unusual in the science of stem cell research. After all, it was experiments on the most obscure animals—newts, flatworms, earthworms, hydras, and roundworms—that first opened the door to regenerative medicine. Those first simple experiments have led to one of medicine's most cutting-edge sciences—a science that holds great promise but also numerous mysteries that scientists have yet to unravel.

Source Notes

Introduction: The Potential of Stem Cell Therapy

1. Quoted in Patrick Perry, "Breakthroughs: On the Brink, Turning the Tide on MS," *Saturday Evening Post*, July/August 2009, p. 48.

2. Quoted in CBS News, "Treating MS Symptoms with Stem Cells," February 10, 2009. www.cbsnews.com.

3. Quoted in Perry, "Breakthroughs," p. 49.

4. Quoted in Perry, "Breakthroughs," p. 49.

5. Quoted in CBS News, "Treating MS Symptoms with Stem Cells."

Chapter One: What Are Stem Cells?

6. Lazzaro Spallanzani, *An Essay on Animal Reproductions*. London: T. Becket and P.A. De Hondt, 1769, p. 30.

7. Jay Phelan, *What Is Life? A Guide to Biology*. New York: Freeman, 2010, p. 78.

8. Leo Furcht and William Hoffman, *The Stem Cell Dilemma: Beacons of Hope or Harbingers of Doom?* New York: Arcade, 2008, pp. 38–39.

9. Michael Bellomo, *The Stem Cell Divide: The Facts, the Fiction, and the Fear Driving the Greatest Scientific, Political, and Religious Debate of Our Time*. New York: Amacom, 2006, p. 32.

10. Furcht and Hoffman, *The Stem Cell Dilemma*, p. 41.

11. Quoted in Ann B. Parson, *The Proteus Effect: Stem Cells and Their Promise for Medicine*. Washington, DC: Joseph Henry, 2004, p. 40.

Chapter Two: The Mysteries of Embryonic Stem Cells

12. Quoted in Science Blog, "Former Police Officer Kris Gulden Testifies in Support of Therapeutic Cloning," January 29, 2003. www.scienceblog.com.

13. Quoted in Gregg Easterbrook, "Medical Evolution," *New Republic*, March 10, 1999, p. 20.

14. Quoted in Easterbrook, "Medical Evolution," p. 20.

15. Quoted in Jennifer Heldt Powell, "Cultivating a Breakthrough," *Boston Herald*, November 9, 1998, p. 35.

16. Quoted in CNN, "Obama Overturns Bush Policy on Stem Cells," March 9, 2009. www.cnn.com.

17. Quoted in J. Travis, "Race to Find Human Stem Cells Ends in Tie," *Science News*, November 7, 1998, p. 293.

18. Quoted in Will Dunham, "Experts Take Heart at Stem Cell Growth," *Adelaide Advertiser* (Australia), August 2, 2001, p. 30.

19. Quoted in Rick Weiss, "Two Studies Bolster Stem Cells' Use in Fighting Disease," *Washington Post*, September 27, 2004, p. A-3.

20. Quoted in Robert Cooke, "Undebatable Promise: Stem Cell Research Advances as Lawmakers Wrangle over Regulation," *Newsday*, August 7, 2001, p. C-3.

21. Quoted in Oliver Burkeman, "Man of Steel," *Guardian*, September 17, 2002. www.guardian.co.uk.

22. Quoted in Karen Kaplan, "Stem Cell Therapy to Be Tested on Spinal Cord Injuries," *Los Angeles Times*, January 24, 2009. http://articles.latimes.com.

23. Quoted in Kate Lunau, "Growing a New Heart," *Maclean's*, March 2, 2009, p. 38.

24. Quoted in *London Daily Mail*, "First Human Stem Cell Trial Using IVF Embryos Will Treat Patients Facing Blindness," November 27, 2009. ww.dailymail.co.uk.

Chapter Three: Rebuilding Damaged Bodies with Adult Stem Cells

25. Quoted in Sarah Baldauf, "Clinical Trials Are Testing Stem Cells as Heart Failure Treatment," *U.S. News & World Report*, August 18, 2009. www.usnews.com.

26. Quoted in Baldauf, "Clinical Trials Are Testing Stem Cells as Heart Failure Treatment."

27. Quoted in Baldauf, "Clinical Trials Are Testing Stem Cells as Heart Failure Treatment."

28. Furcht and Hoffman, *The Stem Cell Dilemma*, p. 39.

29. Cynthia Fox, *Cell of Cells: The Global Race to Capture and Control the Stem Cell*. New York: Norton, 2007, p. 214.

30. Quoted in David Rose, "Diabetics Cured in Stem Cell Treatment Advance," *Times Online*, April 11, 2007. www.timesonline.co.uk.

31. Quoted in *Medical News Today*, "Testing Stem Cells for Peripheral Artery Disease—Indiana University School of Medicine Has Begun Unique Clinical Trial," February 10, 2006. www.medicalnews today.com.

32. Quoted in Anne Marie Tiernon, "Adult Stem Cell Trial Sees Success at IU," Eyewitness News-13, February 2007. www.wthr.com.

33. Quoted in Tiernon, "Adult Stem Cell Trial Sees Success at IU."

34. Quoted in Andrea Gerlin, "The Hard Cell," *Time International*, October 9, 2006, p. 48.

35. Quoted in Gerlin, "The Hard Cell," p. 48.

36. Quoted in Brian Bergman, "Stem Cell Central," *Maclean's*, May 30, 2005, p. 46.

Chapter Four: Therapeutic Cloning: Altering the DNA of Stem Cells

37. Quoted in BBC News, "Cloning Treats Mouse Parkinson's," March 23, 2008. http://news.bbc.co.uk.

38. Peter T. Lansbury and Tom Fagan, "A Fix for Faulty Proteins," *Newsweek*, June 10, 2005. www.newsweek.com.

39. Quoted in Alice Dembner, "First Clone Made of Human Embryo; Critics Decry Work at Worcester Lab," *Boston Globe*, November 26, 2001, p. A-1.

40. Quoted in Lisa Eckelbecker, "Latest Advanced Cell Success Suggests New Stem Cell Option," *Worcester (MA) Telegram & Gazette*, February 1, 2001, p. A-1.

41. Quoted in Daniel Q. Haney, Associated Press, "Therapeutic Cloning Used to Aid Lab Animal," *Albany Times Union*, March 8, 2002, p. A-4.

42. Quoted in Choe-Sang Hun and Nicholas Wade, "Korean Cloning Scientist Quits over Report He Faked His Research," *New York Times*, December 24, 2005, p. A-1.

43. Furcht and Hoffman, *The Stem Cell Dilemma*, p. 40.

44. Quoted in Maggie Fox, Reuters, "Cloned Mice Cells Treat Parkinson's," Australian Broadcasting Corporation, March 24, 2008. www.abc.net.au.

45. Quoted in Mary Duenwald, "A Conversation with Michael J. Fox—a 'Lucky Man' Who Puts His Celebrity to Work," *New York Times*, May 14, 2002, p. F-6.

46. Quoted in BBC News, "Cloning Treats Mouse Parkinson's."

47. Quoted in Pallab Ghosh, "Genetic Advances Raise IVF Hopes," BBC News, August 26, 2009. http://news.bbc.co.uk.

Chapter Five: New Advancements, New Challenges

48. Quoted in Martin Fackler, "Risk Taking Is in His Genes," *New York Times*, December 11, 2007, p. F-1.

49. Quoted in Gina Kolata, "Scientists Bypass Need for Embryo to Get Stem Cells," *New York Times*, November 21, 2007, p. A-1.

50. Furcht and Hoffman, *The Stem Cell Dilemma*, pp. 67–68.

51. Quoted in Kolata, "Scientists Bypass Need for Embryo to Get Stem Cells," p. A-1.

52. Quoted in Kolata, "Scientists Bypass Need for Embryo to Get Stem Cells," p. A-1.

53. Quoted in Alice Park, "Stem Cell Research: The Quest Resumes," *Time*, January 29, 2009. www.time.com.

54. Quoted in Park, "Stem Cell Research."

55. Quoted in John Roach, "Liposuction Fat Turned into Stem Cells, Study Says," *National Geographic*, September 8, 2009. http://news.nationalgeographic.com.

56. Quoted in Roach, "Liposuction Fat Turned into Stem Cells, Study Says."

57. Quoted in David J. Lynch, "Paralysis Patients Take a Chance," *USA Today*, June 20, 2005, p. D-1.

58. Quoted in Lynch, "Paralysis Patients Take a Chance."

59. Quoted in Lynch, "Paralysis Patients Take a Chance."

60. Quoted in Eric Lloyd, "Umbilical Cord Blood: The Future of Stem Cell Research?" *National Geographic*, April 6, 2006. http://news.nationalgeographic.com.

Facts About Stem Cell Research

Stem Cell Lines

• By 2008 the original 64 embryonic stem cell lines created prior to President George W. Bush's federal funding ban had dwindled to 21 due to the exhaustion of the lines.

• By early 2010, after federal funding to embryonic stem cell research had been restored for nearly a year, the number of active stem cell lines stood at 40.

• In order to be regarded as pluripotent, cells in an embryonic stem cell line must continue growing in a laboratory dish without differentiating for at least six months.

• A study by the University of Cambridge concluded that just 150 viable embryonic stem cell lines could provide virtually all the research and therapy needs of Great Britain.

• Scientists at Advanced Cell Technology in Massachusetts have created a stem cell line with a single stem cell withdrawn from a blastocyst containing just eight cells; the Advanced Cell scientists did not destroy the blastocyst by withdrawing that one cell.

Frozen Embryos

• Because the success rate of in vitro fertilization is only 50 percent, in vitro fertilization clinics typically fertilize and freeze many eggs drawn from a patient.

• According to the RAND Corporation, a nonprofit organization that examines public policy issues, there are more than 400,000 embryos sitting in storage in freezers at in vitro fertilization clinics.

- Fewer than 100 Americans have been born from frozen embryos donated to other couples by the parents who provided the fertilized embryos; these children are known as "snowflake babies."

- According to the publication *Gene Therapy*, few embryos donated by in vitro clinics yield viable stem cells; for example, at the Jones Institute, a clinic in Virginia, just 100 of 10,000 frozen embryos in storage are believed capable of providing viable stem cells.

- Since 1978, when the first baby was born through in vitro fertilization, about 3 million babies have been conceived through the technique, according to the European Society of Human Reproduction and Embryology.

- The first stem cell lines created at the University of Wisconsin were drawn from cells contained in 36 frozen embryos; from those embryos, five cell lines were created.

- Of the first five stem cell lines created at the University of Wisconsin, four continued dividing for six months and the fifth continued dividing for two years.

Cell Biology

- Although humans typically have trillions of cells in their bodies, all human cells can be classified into 240 specific types of cells.

- After differentiation, the typical human cell is capable of dividing about 50 times.

- The apparatus in the cell that promotes division is known as the telomere, which protects the cell against the loss of genes. Each time the cell divides, it loses a piece of the telomere. When the telomere is exhausted, the cell dies.

- Embryonic stem cells can divide much more frequently than differentiated cells. Embryonic stem cells can divide between 300 and 450 times in a process that can go on for years.

- Zygotes typically divide on the day after conception, forming two cells. By the next day the zygote has formed eight cells. This stage of embryonic development is known as the morula. By the fifth day the blastocyst has formed, containing 100 or more cells.

Cord Blood and Fetal Tissue Research

- According to the U.S. Food and Drug Administration, 6,000 patients worldwide have been treated with cord blood stem cell transplants.

- Although many political leaders and members of the public oppose research using fetal tissue, experiments on cells drawn from fetal tissue have helped develop vaccines for German measles and chicken pox, according to the U.S. Centers for Disease Control and Prevention.

- Biologists want to study cells in fetal tissue because it is believed that genes responsible for Alzheimer's disease, prostate cancer, and diabetes may be activated during fetal development; therefore fetal stem cells may hold the key for curing those diseases.

- Long before stem cells were drawn out of fetal tissue, doctors transplanted fetal tissue into the spinal cords of paralyzed people in efforts to restore movement in their limbs; such surgeries as well as research into fetal tissue have been legal since 1975.

Human Trials

- In the first human trials involving embryonic stem cells in the United States, researchers plan to monitor the progress of the patients for 15 years. All the patients are paralyzed individuals who will receive injections of 2 million stem cells into their spinal cords.

- The paralyzed patients undergoing the treatments must receive embryonic stem cell injections within 14 days of their accidents; otherwise their spinal cords develop scar tissue that cannot be repaired by stem cells.

- By 2009 about 30,000 Americans had participated in human trials involving injections of adult stem cells.

- Patients who suffer from 72 diseases have been treated with adult stem cells as part of clinical trials.

- In France, researchers plan to begin human trials on a technique that transplants embryonic stem cells into the skin of burn victims to help grow new skin. In the past, physicians have grafted skin from cadavers onto the bodies of people who suffer from severe burns, but this tissue is often rejected by the patients.

- Physicians at Edinburgh University in Scotland have conducted a human trial using adult stem cells drawn from patients to repair their damaged bones and cartilage, which is the spongy tissue found in joints. The physicians who led the trial believe the procedure could eventually replace the need to provide people with artificial hips and knees.

- Researchers at Manchester University in Great Britain have proposed human trials for an embryonic stem cell therapy believed capable of curing baldness caused by a condition known as ectodermal dysplasia. The researchers believe they can coax the stem cells into forming hair follicles.

- By 2010, the U.S. Food and Drug Administration was considering proposals from American biotech companies to approve human trials for embryonic stem cell therapies that would treat Lou Gehrig's disease, diabetes, and macular degeneration, which is a cause of blindness.

Related Organizations

American Society for Reproductive Medicine
1209 Montgomery Hwy.
Birmingham, AL 35216-2809
phone: (205) 978-5000
fax: (205) 978-5005
e-mail: asrm@asrm.org
Web site: www.asrm.org

The society represents physicians who specialize in treating patients who are unable to conceive children. By following the link for frequently asked questions about cloning and stem cells on the organization's Web site, students can find information explaining somatic cell nuclear transfer.

California Institute for Regenerative Medicine
210 King St.
San Francisco, CA 94107
phone: (415) 396-9100
fax: (415) 396-9141
e-mail: info@cirm.ca.gov
Web site: www.cirm.ca.gov

The agency was established to distribute $3 billion in state funds to universities, medical institutions, and private laboratories in California that pursue embryonic stem cell research. By following the "All Funded Grants" link on the agency's Web site, visitors can read descriptions about each project that has received funding from the agency.

Center for iPS Cell Research and Application
53 Kawahara-cho, Shogoin Yoshida
Sakyo-ku, Kyoto 606-8507, Japan

RELATED ORGANIZATIONS

phone: 81-75-751-4842
fax: 81-75-751-0691
e-mail: ips-contact@cira.kyoto-u.ac.jp
Web site: www.cira.kyoto-u.ac.jp/e

The center at Kyoto University houses the research performed by Shinya Yamanaka, a developer of induced pluripotent stem cells (iPS). Students who visit the center's Web site can follow the link to "Resources," which provides basic information on iPS. Students can also view a video, in English, of Yamanaka discussing iPS cells and their significance in stem cell research.

Coalition for the Advancement of Medical Research

2021 K St. NW, Suite 305
Washington, DC 20006
phone: (202) 725-0339
e-mail: CAMResearch@yahoo.com
Web site: www.camradvocacy.org

The coalition is composed of more than 100 universities, medical research institutes, patients' groups, and other advocacy organizations that support embryonic stem cell research. By following the link to "What's New," visitors to the coalition's Web site can read an archive of news stories covering the latest advances in the science.

Do No Harm: The Coalition of Americans for Research Ethics

1100 H St. NW, Suite 700
Washington, DC 20005
phone: (202) 347-6840
fax: (202) 347-6849
Web site: www.stemcellresearch.org

The coalition has compiled many resources supporting its position that viable alternatives to embryonic stem cell research are available. Students who visit the group's Web site can find news articles on adult stem cells as well as induced pluripotent stem cells, download government reports by the Bush administration's President's Council on Bioethics, and read transcripts of testimony by experts who testified about adult stem cell research before Congress.

Family Research Council

801 G St. NW
Washington, DC 20001
phone: (800) 225-4008
Web site: www.frc.org

The Family Research Council opposes embryonic stem cell research but endorses research involving adult stem cells and induced pluripotent stem cells. By following the link to "Stem Cells and Biotechnology," students who visit the council's Web site can find many essays written by council officials explaining their positions.

Genetics Policy Institute

11924 Forest Hill Blvd., Suite 22
Wellington, FL 33414-6258
phone: (888) 238-1423
fax: (561) 791-3889
Web site: www.genpol.org

The institute promotes stem cell research and sponsors the annual World Stem Cell Summit, which features speeches by experts as well as panel discussions that endorse expanding the research. Visitors to the organization's Web site can download the *World Stem Cell* report, providing updates on research into regenerative medicine.

Harvard Stem Cell Institute

42 Church St.
Cambridge, MA 02138
phone: (617) 496-4050
e-mail: hsci@harvard.edu
Web site: www.hsci.harvard.edu

The Harvard University Stem Cell Institute explores cutting-edge stem cell science. By following the Web site's links to "Public & Press," students can find an overview of stem cell science, including many updates on the development of induced pluripotent stem cells.

National Institutes of Health

9000 Rockville Pike
Bethesda, MD 20892

phone: (301) 496-4000
e-mail: NIHinfo@od.nih.gov
Web site: www.nih.gov

The National Institutes of Health is the federal government's chief funding arm for medical research projects. The agency plans to spend billions of dollars on embryonic stem cell research. Students can find an explanation of the science behind stem cell research by accessing the agency's Web site at http://stemcells.nih.gov/index.asp.

New York Stem Cell Foundation
163 Amsterdam Ave., Box 309
New York, NY 10023
phone: (212) 787-4111
e-mail: Info@NYSCF.org
Web site: www.nyscf.org

The foundation raises funds for stem cell research and sponsors public information programs and conferences. The site's link to "Stem Cells 101" provides information on stem cell research. The foundation's newsletter, which can be downloaded, contains news stories and updates on developments in the field.

University of Wisconsin Stem Cell and Regenerative Medicine Center
5009 WIMR, 1111 Highland Ave.
Madison, WI 53705
phone: (608) 265-8668
fax: (608) 263-5267
Web site: http://stemcells.wisc.edu/contact.html

The University of Wisconsin laboratory, headed by stem cell pioneer James A. Thomson, is responsible for some of the major advancements in the science, including the first extraction of stem cells from embryos donated by in vitro fertilization clinics. By following the links on the center's Web site for "Newsroom," students can find updates on the center's latest research projects.

Books

Charles E. Dinsmore, ed., *A History of Regeneration Research: Milestones in the Evolution of a Science.* Cambridge, England: Cambridge University Press, 2008.

Cynthia Fox, *Cell of Cells: The Global Race to Capture and Control the Stem Cell.* New York: Norton, 2007.

Lauri S. Friedman and Hal Marcovitz, *Is Stem Cell Research Necessary?* San Diego, CA: ReferencePoint Press, 2010.

Leo Furcht and William Hoffman, *The Stem Cell Dilemma: Beacons of Hope or Harbingers of Doom?* New York: Arcade, 2008.

Margaret Haerens, ed., *At Issue: Embryonic and Adult Stem Cells.* Farmington Hills, MI: Greenhaven Press, 2009.

Periodicals

Sarah Baldauf, "Clinical Trials Are Testing Stem Cells as Heart Failure Treatment," *U.S. News & World Report,* Aug. 18, 2009.

Gina Kolata, "Scientists Bypass Need for Embryo to Get Stem Cells," *New York Times,* November 21, 2007.

Kate Lunau, "Growing a New Heart," *Maclean's,* March 2, 2009.

Patrick Perry, "Breakthroughs: On the Brink, Turning the Tide on MS," *Saturday Evening Post,* July–August 2009.

Rita Rubin, "Paralysis Doesn't Preclude Action for Ex-Police Officer; Now Kris Gulden Is a Teacher and Stem Cell Activist," *USA Today,* April 21, 2009.

Web Sites

Christopher & Dana Reeve Foundation (www.christopherreeve.org). This research and advocacy foundation's site includes many resources on stem cell research, which was promoted by the late actor following the riding accident that left him paralyzed. Students can find transcripts of the actor's testimony before Congress, urging lawmakers to approve funding for embryonic stem cell research.

Michael J. Fox Foundation (www.michaeljfox.org). Established by the actor, who has been diagnosed with Parkinson's disease, the Web site provides updates on scientific research projects, many of which employ stem cells. By following the link to "Living with Parkinson's," students can find explanations of the disease and how it manifests itself in symptoms that rob people of their ability to speak while suffering from tremors and rigid muscles.

NOVA, **"Stem Cells"** (www.pbs.org/wgbh/nova/sciencenow/3209/04. html). Students visiting the Web site sponsored by the PBS series *NOVA* can find many resources on adult and embryonic stem cells as well as therapeutic cloning. The site also covers the political fight to approve federal funding for embryonic stem cell research in the United States, including the restrictions placed on research and funding by the Dickey-Wicker Amendment and by former President George W. Bush.

On Being a Scientist: A Guide to Responsible Conduct in Research (www.nap.edu/openbook.php?record_id=12192&page=R1). This is a free, downloadable book from the National Academy of Sciences Committee on Science, Engineering, and Public Policy. The 2009 edition provides a clear explanation of the responsible conduct of scientific research. Chapters on treatment of data, mistakes and negligence, the scientist's role in society, and other topics offer invaluable insight for student researchers.

United Kingdom Stem Cell Foundation, "Stem Cell Research" (http://domain883347.sites.fasthosts.com/research/index.html). The foundation supporting stem cell research in Great Britain provides a background on the history and science behind the research. By accessing the link for "Research Presentation," students can view an animation that addresses specific diseases that stem cell therapy may cure, including blindness, stroke, Parkinson's disease, and diabetes.

Washington Post, **"On Faith: The (Im)Morality of Stem Cell Research"** (http://newsweek.washingtonpost.com/onfaith/2009/03/ embryonic_stem_cell_research/all.html). The *Washington Post* has posted written comments by 20 political leaders, theologians, scientists, and other experts stating their positions in support and opposition to using stem cells drawn from human embryos for medical research.

Index

therapeutic, hurdles in, 56–57

See also somatic cell nuclear transfer

congestive heart failure, 12

treatment by stem cell therapy, 47–48

cord blood stem cells, 18

definition of, 72

harvesting of, 23 (illustration)

coronary artery, blocked, 47 (illustration)

Crick, Francis, 51

Crohn's disease, 12

Daley, George Q., 55

Darwin, Charles, 51

de Réaumur, Rene-Antoine Ferchault, 15

diabetes, type 1, stem cell therapy for, 45–46

Dickey, Jay, 31

Dickey-Wicker Amendment (1995), 31

differentiation

of cells, 16

spontaneous, tumor formation and, 21

of stem cells, 19

Diggs, Ruth, 46, 49

DNA (deoxyribonucleic acid), 19

discovery of structure of, 51

in SCNT, 52

Dolly the sheep, 56

Driesch, Hans, 16

embryo, 17, 29

removal of cells from blastocyst kills, 30

embryonic stem cell research, ban on federal funding of, 29–31

embryonic stem cells, 19

adult stem cells *vs.*, 44

definition of, 26

differention of, into heart cells, 33–34

Evans, Martin, 27, 35

Evans, Robert, 27

eye cells, creation

from iPS cells, 67

from stem cells, 38

Fagan, Tom, 52

fetal tissue, definition of, 69

Food and Drug Administration, U.S. (FDA), 12, 26

Fost, Norman, 32

Fox, Cynthia, 45

Fox, Michael J., 59

Furcht, Leo, 19, 22, 43, 58, 64

Furton, Edward, 30

gametes (germ cell lines), definition of, 28

Gearhart, John D., 28, 29, 31, 36

Gebbie, Kristine, 72

Gelsinger, Jesse, 66

genes, definition of, 59

Picture Credits

Cover: iStockphoto.com
AP Images: 27, 63
iStockphoto.com: 8 (upper right)
Landov: 57
Photos.com: 8 (lower left), 9
Science Photo Library: 11, 13, 18, 23, 30, 37, 42, 47, 53, 70

PICTURE CREDITS

About the Author

Hal Marcovitz has written more than 150 books for young readers. A former daily newspaper reporter and columnist, he makes his home in Chalfont, Pennsylvania, with his wife, Gail, and daughter, Ashley. As a journalist, Marcovitz is a three-time winner of the Keystone Press Award, the Pennsylvania Newspaper Association's highest award for journalism. His 2005 biography of U.S. House Speaker Nancy Pelosi was named to *Booklist* magazine's list of recommended feminist books for young readers. He also served as chief writer and associate editor for *Taught to Lead,* an anthology of essays chronicling the educations of the presidents of the United States, and is coauthor of *Bloom's Literary Places: Rome,* a traveler's guide to places in Rome where famous writers such as F. Scott Fitzgerald, Tennessee Williams, and Gore Vidal lived and worked. Marcovitz is also the author of the comic novel *Painting the White House.*

ABOUT THE AUTHOR